Prentice Hall's

question and answer review

of Health Information Management

8th EDITION

Susan Pritchard Bailey, MBA, RRA

Michelle A. Green, MPS, RRA, CMA
State University of New York
College of Technology
Alfred, New York

Jennifer A. Gehen, MS, RHIA
Kaleida Health of Buffalo
Children's Hospital of Buffalo
Buffalo, New York

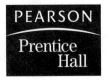

PEARSON
Prentice
Hall

Upper Saddle River, New Jersey 0

Library of Congress Cataloging-in-Publication Data

Bailey, Susan Pritchard.
   Prentice Hall's question and answer review of health information management / Susan Pritchard Bailey, Michelle A. Green, Jennifer A. Gehen.—8th ed.
      p. cm.
   Rev. ed. of: Health information management. 7th ed. c1998.
   Includes bibliographical references.
   ISBN 0-13-098257-1
   1. Medical records—Management—Examinations, questions, etc.
   [DNLM: 1. Medical Records—Examination Questions. 2. Forms and Records Control—methods—Examination Questions. 3. Information Management—methods—Examination
Questions. 4. Medical Records Systems, Computerized—Examination Questions. WX 18.2 B156p 2005] I. Title: Question and answer review of health information management.
II. Green, Michelle A. III. Gehen, Jennifer A. IV. Bailey, Susan Pritchard. Health information management. V. Prentice-Hall, inc. VI. Title.

RA976.B35 2005
651.5'04261'076—dc22

                                                                                                                          2004004852

Publisher: *Julie Levin Alexander*
Publisher's Assistant: *Regina Bruno*
Acquisitions Editor: *Joan Gill*
Associate Editor: *Melissa Kerian*
Editorial Assistant: *Jaquay Felix*
Director of Manufacturing and Production: *Bruce Johnson*
Managing Editor for Production: *Patrick Walsh*
Production Liaison: *Cathy O'Connell*
Production Editor: *Patty Donovan, Pine Tree Composition*
Manufacturing Manager: *Ilene Sanford*
Manufacturing Buyer: *Pat Brown*
Creative Director: *Cheryl Asherman*
Senior Design Coordinator: *Christopher Weigand*
Cover and Interior Designer: *Janice Bielawa*
Director of Marketing/Marketing Manager: *Karen Allman*
Channel Marketing Manager: *Rachele Strober*
Marketing Coordinator: *Janet Ryerson*
Media Editor: *John Jordan*
Media Production Manager: *Amy Peltier*
Media Project Manager: *Stephen Hartner*
Composition: *Pine Tree Composition, Inc.*
Printer/Binder: *The Banta Company, VA*
Cover Printer: *Phoenix Color Corp.*

NOTICE

The author and the publisher of this volume have taken care to make certain that the doses of drugs and schedules of treatment are correct and compatible with the standards generally accepted at the time of publication. Nevertheless, as new information becomes available, changes in treatment and in the use of drugs become necessary. The reader is advised to carefully consult the instruction and information material included in the package insert of each drug or therapeutic agent before administration. This advice is especially important when using new or infrequently used drugs. The author and publisher disclaim all responsibility for any liability, loss, injury, or damage incurred as a consequence, directly or indirectly, of the use and application of any of the contents of the volume.

Pearson Education LTD
Pearson Education Australia PTY., Limited
Pearson Education Singapore, Pte. Ltd
Pearson Education North Asia Ltd
Pearson Education, Canada, Ltd

Pearson Educación de Mexico, S.A. de C.V.
Pearson Education—Japan
Pearson Education Malaysia, Pte. Ltd
Pearson Education, Upper Saddle River, New Jersey

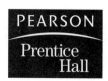

10 9 8 7 6 5 4 3 2 1
ISBN 0-13-098257-1

Contents

Preface / ii
Acknowledgments / iii
Introduction / iv

1 Health Data Content and Structure / 1
2 Health Care Delivery Systems / 19
3 Classification Systems / 35
4 Reimbursement Methodologies / 55
5 ICD-9-CM and CPT-4 Coding / 67
6 Statistics and Data Literacy / 93
7 Legal and Ethical Issues / 109
8 Information Technology / 123
9 Quality Assessment and Performance Improvement / 137
10 Organization and Supervision / 151
11 Human Resources / 171
12 Biomedical Sciences / 189

References / 203
Index / 205

Preface

Prentice Hall's Question and Answer Review of Health Information Management, 8th Edition includes multiple-choice questions, covering material likely to be seen on the RHIA/RHIT exams. The chapters in the book are broken down into content areas as reflected in the RHIA/RHIT examinations. This book is an excellent resource for preparing for the RHIA/RHIT exam. It has been designed to act as a study companion for those who are (1) preparing for the RHIA exam or (2) preparing for the RHIT exam and/or (3) pursuing self-assessment in the health information technology/management field.

The book contains over 850 multiple-choice questions as a means to the overall review of the health information management field. The chapters in this book are arranged by content area as reflected in the RHIA/RHIT Examination Content Outline and AHIMA's latest model curriculum. What is new about the 8th edition is the incorporation of *application and analysis questions* as opposed to primarily *recall-based questions.* The RHIA/RHIT examination questions consist of cognitive skills needed to answer the questions, including ***Recall-RE:***, the ability to recall previously memorized knowledge skills and facts; ***Application-AP:***, the ability to apply recalled knowledge in verbal and written skills; and ***Analysis-AN:***, the ability to apply recalled knowledge in solving a problem or case situation. Therefore, practicing a variety of different knowledge-level questions will be crucial to your success on the exam.

Prentice Hall's Question and Answer Review of Health Information Management, 8th Edition contains 12 chapters. Chapter 1 is Health Data Content and Structure, Chapter 2 is Healthcare Delivery Systems, Chapter 3 is Classification Systems, Chapter 4 is Reimbursement Methodologies, Chapter 5 is ICD-9-CM and CPT-4 Coding, Chapter 6 is Statistics and Data Literacy, Chapter 7 is Legal and Ethical Issues, Chapter 8 is Information Technology, Chapter 9 is Quality Assessment and Performance Improvement, Chapter 10 is Organization and Supervision, Chapter 11 is Human Resources Management, and Chapter 12 is Biomedical Sciences. Each chapter has chapter objectives included to serve as a guide to measure your strengths and weaknesses in the various HIA/HIT content areas. Chapter 11, Human Resources Management, is a unique chapter in that it is geared specifically for RHIA students. However, that doesn't mean that RHIT students shouldn't give these questions a try!

The correct answers and rationales are provided to give students not only the correct answer but also the reasons why the incorrect answers are incorrect. Correct answers are referenced to a primary and secondary text so students can focus their studying on their problem areas.

After reviewing the multiple-choice questions and answers, the reader can practice taking a mock examination provided on the accompanying CD-ROM. The enclosed CD-ROM provides 200 questions with rationales and answers for further study.

There are many uses for this book. This book has been designed to be used for (1) the classroom as a resource for instructors, (2) the RHIA examination, (3) the RHIT examination, and (4) the experienced HIM professional for self-assessment. This book should prove to be a valuable resource for you not only to prepare for an upcoming exam, which will identify strengths and weaknesses, but also will sharpen your health information management skills.

Jennifer A. Gehen, MS, RHIA

Acknowledgments

The following people have been instrumental in this book's publication. I wish to thank them all.

My husband, Erik, whom I dearly love, and whose patience, support, and encouragement during the preparation of this project has been absolutely amazing.

My daughter Casey, who is my pride and joy, the love of my life.

My Mom and Dad, Mom, my best friend and #1 fan, and Dad, thank you for your words of wisdom and spiritual guidance.

In memory of Susan Pritchard Bailey who had given me this wonderful opportunity.

Introduction

 SUCCESS ACROSS THE BOARDS: THE PRENTICE HALL HEALTH REVIEW SERIES

Prentice Hall is pleased to present our review series, **Success Across the Boards.** These authoritative texts give you expert help in preparing for certifying examinations. Each title in the series comes with its own technology package, including a CD-ROM and a Companion Website. You will find that this powerful combination of text and media provides you with expert help and guidance for achieving success across the boards.

COMPONENTS OF THE SERIES:

The series is made up of a book and CD combination.

About the Book

- **Content Review:** Content Areas that may be covered on the RHIA and RHIT examinations are included in this book. This book has been designed to help the student prepare for the RHIA/RHIT certification exams. Over 850 multiple-choice questions are organized by all the topics covered on the RHIA and RHIT exams and follow the exam format to a large extent. Working through these questions will help you assess your strengths and weaknesses in each topic of study. There are different levels of questions consisting of cognitive levels needed to answer the questions provided in each chapter
- **Chapter Objectives:** Each chapter includes objectives, which allow you to preview the topics covered and identify the information and skills you are responsible for knowing.
- **Answers and Rationales:** The correct answer and a rationale for it are given for each question. Rationales for each incorrect answer are provided as well so that you may learn why an answer is incorrect.
- **References:** Answers are referenced to appropriate page numbers in the reference list located in the back of this book. The majority of the questions are referenced to textbooks familiar to HIT and HIA students that are Abdelhak's *HEALTH INFORMATION: Management of a Strategic Resource* and *John's Health Information*

Management Technology. However, there are other numerous resources that are included to assist the reader.

About the CD-ROM

A CD-ROM is included in the back of this book. The CD provides additional practice multiple-choice questions with answers, rationales, and references that follow all questions. You will receive immediate feedback to identify your strengths and weaknesses.

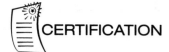

CERTIFICATION

The sponsoring association of RHIA and RHIT certification is the American Health Information Management Association (AHIMA). AHIMA sponsors five certifications: the Registered Health Information Administrator (RHIA); the Registered Health Information Technician (RHIT); the Certified Coding Specialist-Hospital-based (CCS); the Certified Coding Specialist-Physician-based (CCS-P); and the Certified Coding Associate (CCA).

Registered Health Information Administrator (RHIA) Eligibility Requirements:

To be eligible for RHIA certification, an individual must meet one of the following eligibility requirements:

- Have a baccalaureate degree from a CAAHEP-accredited health information administration (HIA) program; or
- Have a baccalaureate degree from an accredited college or university and a certificate in HIA from a CAAHEP-accredited program; or
- Have a degree from an HIA baccalaureate degree program in a foreign country whose professional association has an agreement of reciprocity with AHIMA; or
- Be an RHIT who meets the conditions of the Proviso to the *Standards for Initial Certification for Registered Health Information Administrators* approved by the 1998 AHIMA House of Delegates for RHIA initial certifications awarded January 1, 1999, through December 31, 2004. These conditions are as follows:

a. Have a baccalaureate degree or higher from an accredited institution of post-secondary education; and
b. Have received RHIT certification on or before December 31, 1999; and
c. Have complied with the *Standards for Maintenance of Registered Health Information Technician (RHIT) Certification* (RHIA/RHIT Certification Guide, p. 4).

Registered Health Information Technician (RHIT) Eligibility Requirements:

To be eligible for RHIT certification, an individual must meet one of the following eligibility requirements:

- Have an associate's degree from a CAAHEP-accredited health information technology program (HIT); or
- Have a degree from an HIT associate's degree program in a foreign country whose professional association has an agreement of reciprocity with AHIMA; or
- Have a certification in health information technology from the AHIMA Independent Study Program (ISP), 30 semester (45 quarter) hours of college credit from an accredited college or university, and have completed ISP course requirements as specified at the time of enrollment in the program. Beginning in September 2002, individuals must earn an associate's degree in addition to completing the Independent Study Program in order to be eligible to take the RHIT exam (RHIA/RHIT Certification Guide, p. 4).

ABOUT THE EXAM

The RHIA and RHIT examinations are a written test administered by the Applied Measurement Professionals, Inc. (AMP). AMP is under contract to AHIMA to help develop, administer, and score the RHIA and RHIT examinations.

The examinations are administered daily via computer at AMP Assessment Centers geographically distributed throughout the United States. The exam appointments are scheduled on a first-come, first-serve basis. A complete listing of Assessment Centers can be found on AMP's Web site at www.goamp.com. The RHIA exam consists of 160 questions. The RHIT exam consists of 130 questions.

Information about examinations may change, so be sure to obtain the RHIA/RHIT Certification Guide, which contains the application and instructions. You may download the application from AHIMA's website by going to www.ahima.org. For information about AHIMA's certification programs, or for information about the RHIA and RHIT exams, contact:

American Health Information Management
    Association
Attn: RHIA/RHIT Examination
233 N. Michigan Ave., Suite 2150
Chicago, IL 60601-5800
Telephone: (312) 233-1100
Fax: (312) 233-1090
E-mail: certdept@ahima.org
Web Site: www.ahima.org

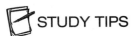 STUDY TIPS

Review Materials

Choose review materials that contain the information you need to study. Save time by making sure that you aren't studying anything you don't need to. The best preparation before the exam is to work through the questions in this review book to determine your strengths and weaknesses. The page references at the end of each answer will direct you to familiar textbooks so that you can obtain additional information on the question topic.

Set a Study Schedule

Use your time management skills to set a schedule that will help you feel as prepared as you can be. Consider all the relevant factors: the materials you need to study; how many months, weeks, or days until the test date; and how much time you can study each day. If you establish your schedule ahead of time and write it in your date book, you will be much more likely to follow it.

Take Practice Tests

Practice as much as possible, using the questions in this book, on the accompanying CD-ROM, and on the companion website. These questions were designed to follow the format of questions that appear on the exam you will take, so the more you practice with these questions, the better prepared you will be on test day. For best results, we recommend that you take a practice test 2 to 3 weeks before you are scheduled to take the actual exam. Spend the next weeks targeting the areas in which you performed poorly and practice additional questions in those areas.

Practice under test-like conditions: in a quiet room, with no books or notes to help you when appropriate and use coding books only when asked, and with a clock telling you when to quit. Try to come as close as you can to duplicating the actual test situation.

TAKING THE EXAMINATION

Prepare Physically

When taking the exam, you need to work efficiently under time pressure. If your body is tired or under stress, you might not think as clearly or perform as well as you usually do. If you can, avoid staying up all night. Get some sleep so that you can wake up rested and alert.

Eating right is also important. The best advice is to eat a light, well-balanced meal before a test. When time is short, grab a quick energy snack such as a banana, orange juice, or a granola bar.

The Examination Site

The examination site must be located before the required examination time. One suggestion is to find the site and parking facilities the day before the test. Parking fee information should be obtained ahead of time so that sufficient money can be taken along on the examination day.

Allow plenty of time for travel to the site in case of unexpected mishaps such as traffic snarls. During travel, think positive thoughts (e.g., "My preparation for the exam was thorough, so I'll be able to answer the questions easily"). Maintain a confident attitude to prevent unnecessary stress.

Materials

Be sure to take all required identified materials, registration forms, and any other items required by the testing organization or center. Thoroughly read information and instructions supplied by the testing organizations to be sure you have all necessary materials before the day of the exam.

Read Test Directions

Read the examination directions thoroughly! Because some board examinations have different test sections directions, it is important to be aware of changes in directions. Read each set of directions completely before starting a new section of questions.

Machine-scored tests require that you use a special pencil to fill in a small box on a computerized answer sheet. Use the right pencil (usually a number 2) and mark your answers in the correct space. Neatness counts on these tests, because the computer can misread stray pencil marks or partially erased answers. Periodically, check the answer number against the question number to make sure they match. One question skipped can cause every answer following it to be marked incorrect. Your examination may also be administered via computer, which will be mentioned later.

Selecting the Right Answer

Keep in mind that only one answer is correct. First read the stem of the question with *each* possible choice provided, and eliminate choices that are obviously incorrect. Be cautious about choosing the fist answer that *might* be correct; all possibilities should be considered before the final choice is made; the best answer should be selected.

IF a question is complicated, try to break it down into small sections that are easy to understand. Pay special attention to qualifiers such as *only, except,* and the like. For example, negative words in a question can confuse your understanding of what the question asks ("Which of the following is *not* . . .").

Intelligent Guessing

If you don't know the answer, eliminate those answers that you know or suspect are wrong. Your goal is to narrow down your choices. Here are some questions to ask yourself:

- Is the choice accurate in its own terms? If there is an error in the choice—for example, a term that is incorrectly defined—the answer is wrong.

- Is the choice relevant? An answer may be accurate, but it might not relate to the essence of the question.
- Are there any qualifiers, such as *always, never, all, none,* or *every?* Qualifiers make it easy to find an exception that makes a choice incorrect.

Mark answers you aren't sure of, and go back to them at the end of the test.

As yourself whether you would make the same guesses again. Chances are that you will leave your answers alone, but you may notice something that will make you change your mind—a qualifier that affects meaning or a remembered fact that will enable you to answer the question without guessing.

Watch the Clock

Keep track of how much time is left and how you are progressing. Wear a watch or bring a small clock with you to the test room. A wall clock may be broken, or there may be no clock at all.

Some students are so concerned about time that they rush through the exam and have time left over. In such situations, it's easy to leave early. The best approach, however, is to take your time. Stay until the end so that you can check your answers.

Computerized Exams

To ensure that you are comfortable with the computer test format, be sure to practice on the computer using the CD-ROM that is included in the back of this book.

Since certification exam requirements vary, it is important to determine before taking a computerized exam whether you can change your answer after you strike a key for a particular answer. Checking your answers is a very important part of taking a major certification exam. Thus do not enter an answer on a computerized exam unless you (1) have the option to change it as you are checking your answers or (2) are absolutely certain that your answer is correct when you first enter it.

During the exam, check the computer screen after an answer is entered to verify that the answer appears as it was entered. If you feel fatigued, close your eyes, take a few deep breaths, and stretch your arms and shoulders; then resume the examination.

KEY TO SUCCESS ACROSS THE BOARD

- Study, review, and practice
- Keep a positive, confident attitude
- Follow all directions on the examination
- Do your best

Good luck!

You are encouraged to visit **http://www. pren-hall.com/success** *for additional tips on studying, test taking, and other keys to success. At this stage of your education and career, you will find these tips helpful.*

Some of the study and test-taking tips were adapted from Keys to Effective Learning, Second Edition, by Carol Carter, Joyce Bishop, and Sarah Lyman Kravits.

1

Health Data Content and Structure

objectives

After completion of this chapter, the student will be able to:

- ➤ Describe the documentation requirements of the health record.

- ➤ Discuss the structure and content of the health record.

- ➤ Identify the different data sets utilized in health care organizations.

- ➤ Describe the indexes and registries utilized in health care.

- ➤ Differentiate between primary versus secondary records.

- ➤ Explain the principles of paper-based and computer-based forms design and analysis.

- ➤ Perform quantitative and qualititative analysis on health records.

- ➤ Explain the importance of appropriate documentation and related issues.

- ➤ Describe the different filing systems utilized in health care.

- ➤ Discuss health information retention and retrieval issues.

DIRECTIONS (Questions 1–81): Each of the questions or incomplete statements below is followed by suggested answers or completions. Select the **best** answer in each case.

---

1. Which was the first major U.S. impetus for improving hospital health records?
   A. organization of the American Health Information Management Association
   B. establishment of the JCAHO's numerous accreditation programs
   C. opening of the first incorporated hospital, known as Pennsylvania Hospital
   D. creation of the American College of Surgeons' hospital standardization program

2. A rubber stamp of Dr. Day's signature is acceptable for use if
   A. it is stored in the health information department and is used only by Dr. Day
   B. it is used by Dr. Day and her clinical staff because she gave them permission to do so
   C. Dr. Day signed a statement regarding its use; the statement is stored with the facility's administration
   D. it is utilized only by Dr. Day and the other physicians involved in her group practice

3. The integrated health record format is identified by its
   A. arrangement according to the source of the information
   B. association of treatment and therapies with patient problems
   C. organization of reports in strict chronological date order
   D. standardized forms as recommended by the JCAHO

4. Regulations about physician completion of health records are developed by the
   A. health information management department
   B. acute care facility's medical staff

   C. health care facility's governing body
   D. hospital's administrative offices

5. Which would be considered a primary record?
   A. diagnostic index that contains ICD-9-CM codes on Sally Smith
   B. utilization review committee minutes concerning patient Sally Smith
   C. Sally Smith's emergency department record dated January 1
   D. emergency department log containing a January 1 entry for Sally Smith

6. Which of the following demonstrates the personal use of the health record?
   A. information from Sally Smith's record included in a hospital statistical report
   B. JCAHO survey of 100 records, including that of Sally Smith
   C. quality assurance study that contains information from Sally Smith's record
   D. malpractice case brought to trial that includes Sally Smith's record as evidence

7. Susan is a nurse who brings to your attention an error in the health record. She is uncertain how to make the correction. What would Susan's first step be in amending an error in a health record?
   A. drawing a single line through the error
   B. obliterating the incorrect documentation
   C. documenting the reason for the error
   D. obtaining the supervisor's co-signature

8. A final progress note may be substituted for a discharge summary when a (an)
   A. patient's hospitalization is under 48 hours' duration with minor problems

B. circumcised newborn who develops an infection is discharged within 48 hours

C. obstetrical patient delivers a healthy female newborn via cesarean section

D. expected death of a terminal patient occurs within 48 hours of admission

9. The reanalysis of health records refers to

A. analysis after health providers have worked on records, but prior to permanent filing

B. the assembly of the health record upon receipt from the facility's nursing units

C. authentication of incomplete health records after initial analysis has been done

D. computerized abstracting of health records after the provider has completed them

10. Reports that summarize administration of therapeutic radiation are documented

A. at the conclusion of the administration of each radiation therapy session

B. on a weekly basis, summarizing several radiation therapies administered

C. by the practitioner administering the radiation therapy, at least monthly

D. at the end of the therapeutic radiation treatment for the particular patient

11. A postanesthesia evaluation is documented in the patient's record by the practitioner administering the anesthetic

A. immediately upon conclusion of the surgery

B. within 24 hours after the surgery is performed

C. within 48 hours after the surgery is performed

D. and authenticated by the patient's surgeon

12. The major advantages of the problem-oriented health record include all of the following EXCEPT:

A. it requires the attending physician to consider all of the patient's problems

B. it is easily accepted by physicians, nurses, and allied health professionals

C. it clearly indicates the goals and methods of the physician in treating the patient

D. it allows physicians and others to follow the course of any one problem more easily

13. The master patient index should be kept

A. for 25 years

B. for 10 years

C. for 5 years

D. permanently

14. With alphabetical filing, which of the following names would be filed first?

A. S. Peter Jones

B. Steven Peter Jones

C. Stephen Peter Jones

D. S. Jones

15. Divorce complicates which type of numbering system?

A. social security

B. family

C. unit

D. serial-unit

16. Which system makes it easiest to purge records for microfilming?

A. terminal digit filing

B. serial-unit numbering

C. unit numbering

D. straight numeric filing

17. Which would be considered a major component of the record control function?

A. requisition slip

B. master patient index

C. number index

D. file shelving

18. Which represents records filed within a primary section in terminal digit order?
    A. 00-00-52, 01-00-52, 02-00-52, 03-00-52
    B. 00-00-52, 00-00-53, 00-00-54, 00-00-55
    C. 00-00-52, 01-00-53, 02-00-54, 03-00-55
    D. 00-01-52, 00-02-53, 00-03-54, 00-04-55

19. Which would be the chief criterion for determining record inactivity?
    A. statute of limitations for the state in which health records are generated
    B. amount of space available for efficient storage of newer health records
    C. number of filing personnel available to effectively retrieve or refile records
    D. equipment used to store records in the health information department

20. The terminal digit file area requires 2000 file guides. What is the pattern of file guides?
    A. 00-00-00, 00-05-00, 00-10-00, 00-15-00
    B. 00-00-00, 00-50-00, 01-00-00, 01-50-00
    C. 00-00-00, 00-00-05, 00-00-10, 00-00-15
    D. 00-00-00, 00-00-50, 00-01-00, 00-01-50

21. The four major sections of a problem-oriented health record are
    A. database, problem list, initial plans, progress notes
    B. problem list, SOAP notes, nursing notes, graphic sheets
    C. history and physical, problem list, SOAP notes, resume
    D. initial plans, problem list, SOAP notes, nursing notes

22. The inpatient's record generally begins in the
    A. facility's admitting department
    B. attending physician's office
    C. hospital nursing station
    D. preadmission testing department

23. Which of the following would be found in a history report?
    A. review of systems
    B. differential diagnosis
    C. blood pressure and pulse
    D. the patient's appearance

24. The diagnosis recorded at the conclusion of the history and physical is the
    A. provisional diagnosis
    B. principal diagnosis
    C. primary diagnosis
    D. chief complaint

25. Color coding of health record folders helps prevent
    A. misnumbering of health records
    B. misfiling of health record folders
    C. misinterpretation of record content
    D. misplacement of forms in the record

26. Which organizations' directives establish minimum contents of a health record?
    A. JCAHO, state licensing regulations, Conditions of Participation
    B. state health department rules, Conditions of Participation, JCAHO
    C. conditions of Participation, JCAHO, Memo of Understanding
    D. state licensing regulations, JCAHO, Memo of Understanding

27. Progress notes
    A. are to be documented at least once daily for each patient in the acute care facility
    B. may or may not contain an admission note documented by the attending physician
    C. include a discharge note that is documented at the conclusion of the patient's stay
    D. should consist of information documented in the history and physical examination

28. Quantitative analysis of the health record would include review for
   A. required authentication of all entries
   B. use of abbreviations on the face sheet
   C. potentially compensable events
   D. consistency in documentation of provider entries

29. An infant's record is
   A. filed with the mother's record only if the infant was a premature newborn
   B. separate from the mother's record and contains a few routine forms and reports
   C. filed with the mother's record if the infant is normal (i.e., healthy newborn)
   D. separate from the mother's record if she experienced no delivery complications

30. If a patient falls while in the hospital, an incident form is generated and
   A. a copy is filed in the patient's health record with the original forwarded to administration
   B. reference is made in the health record that an incident report was generated
   C. documentation of the fall and treatment rendered is recorded in the patient's health record
   D. the risk manager meets with the patient to discuss this potentially compensable event

31. Which filing system organizes records in strict chronological order?
   A. terminal digit
   B. middle digit
   C. straight numeric
   D. serial numeric

32. The major advantage of straight numeric filing is
   A. ease in training of employees who file

B. increase in health record confidentiality
   C. ability to monitor file clerk filing activities
   D. reduction in misfiles of health records

33. The terminal digit number filed first in the following series is
   A. 50-63-24
   B. 75-63-24
   C. 75-61-23
   D. 45-52-24

34. Which would provide a chronological listing of all patient admissions?
   A. master patient index
   B. computer abstracts
   C. patient register
   D. number control log

35. Which type of microfilm has the greatest storage density?
   A. aperture cards
   B. roll film
   C. microfiche
   D. microfilm jackets

36. A cancer registry program must acheive which follow-up rate to receive approval by the American College of Surgeons?
   A. 70%
   B. 80%
   C. 90%
   D. 100%

37. The best application for bar coding in the health information department is
   A. coding diagnoses
   B. medical transcription
   C. quantitative analysis
   D. health record tracking

38. Birth and death certificates should be maintained by the facility
    A. permanently
    B. for 25 years
    C. for 15 years
    D. for 10 years

39. The chief complaint included in a history and physical examination report is a statement made by the
    A. family
    B. nurse
    C. patient
    D. physician

40. Which would be considered an ancillary department?
    A. patient billing/collections
    B. environmental services
    C. biomedical maintenance
    D. clinical laboratory/pathology

41. Which statement would be documented in the physical examination report?
    A. occasional headache
    B. palpable axillary node
    C. history of cholecystectomy
    D. pain in right upper quadrant

42. Which is the most important consideration in designing a form?
    A. spacing needed for typing
    B. purpose and need for it
    C. number of copies included
    D. information to be documented

43. Which is documented in the physical examination report?
    A. review of systems
    B. present illness
    C. general survey
    D. chief complaint

44. All would be contained in the physical examination report EXCEPT:
    A. rebound tenderness
    B. rales and rhonchi
    C. thirst and dizziness
    D. negative Romberg sign

45. Standing orders
    A. must be authenticated by the physician after being filed in the chart
    B. can be excluded from the record if they are posted in the nursing unit
    C. may be presigned by the physician prior to duplicating the orders
    D. need to be signed only if the attending physician alters the orders

46. A hospital administrator requests the health information management department to provide a report detailing the number of incomplete discharged health records during the past 6 months. Such a report would be the result of a (an)
    A. survey of diagnostic and procedural indexes
    B. review of discharge lists for the past six months
    C. analysis of health records for deficiencies
    D. breakdown of records according to entry omissions

47. The JCAHO requires creation of a new record for emergency patients
    A. upon the patient's first visit to the emergency department
    B. each time the patient is seen in the emergency department
    C. when the patient is diagnosed with a different condition
    D. if the patient has changed his or her primary physician

48. The first step in developing a problem-oriented record is
    A. obtaining a patient database
    B. documenting the problem list
    C. recording SOAP progress notes
    D. writing initial plans for the patient

49. The *P* in the SOAP note of the problem-oriented record refers to the
    A. patient's progress that has been demonstrated in response to treatment
    B. diagnostic, therapeutic, and educational plans that are being developed
    C. documentation of a particular problem in the patient's progress note
    D. physical assessment conducted on the patient and documented

50. Patients admitted to the hospital on September 18th were issued the following patient numbers: 9010, 2053, 9011, 9012, 3155, 0381. Which numbering system is being used?
    A. serial
    B. unit
    C. serial-unit
    D. terminal digit

51. Which modification of the unit numbering system includes pseudonumbers?
    A. family numbering
    B. serial-unit numbering
    C. serial numbering
    D. social security numbering

52. Unitized microforms include all of the following EXCEPT:
    A. jackets
    B. ultrafiche
    C. rotary
    D. microfiche

53. A disease index organizes patient data according to the

A. classification system used by the facility
B. numbering system used by the facility
C. filing system used by the facility
D. registration method used by the facility

54. How long should annual statistical reports based on monthly analyses of hospital services be kept?
    A. permanently
    B. 25 years
    C. 10 years
    D. 5 years

55. How would the last name, St. John, be filed in an alphabetical file?
    A. St. John
    B. Stjohn
    C. John, St.
    D. Saint John

56. Anytown Medical Center uses a decentralized system for record keeping. The next number in the serial system for inpatient hospital admissions is 16888. The next number to be assigned in the outpatient clinic is unit number 17845. Mary Jones's last number on outpatient admission was 10921 and on hospital admission was 15824. What patient number will be assigned to Mary Jones if she returns to the hospital as an outpatient?
    A. 10921
    B. 17845
    C. 16888
    D. 10922

57. Which number was most recently assigned to a new patient by the admitting department of a facility that uses unit numbering to assign numbers and terminal digit filing to file records?
    A. 44 10 76
    B. 76 02 76
    C. 56 00 76
    D. 89 03 76

58. Inpatient discharges total 1,763 in one month; 521 of these discharged health records are complete at discharge. Calculate the month's incomplete health record rate.
    A. 3.38%
    B. 29.55%
    C. 70.45%
    D. 76.13%

59. Which best describes the organization of the source-oriented record on the nursing unit?
    A. reports are filed in chronological date order
    B. the forms are in reverse chronological order
    C. the record is integrated regarding reports
    D. it has a goal-oriented format to facilitate treatment

60. Which is the most important use of a number index?
    A. control of patient numbers assigned
    B. planning for patient number assignment
    C. retrieval of records according to patient number
    D. listing of patients and their final diagnoses

61. A department maintains records in hard copy form instead of microfilming; it also has limited space for record storage. Which would the department benefit most from?
    A. movable open shelving units
    B. stationary open shelving units
    C. computerized health record
    D. seven-drawer file cabinets

62. A complete autopsy protocol or report is made part of the health record within
    A. 30 days
    B. 2 weeks
    C. 60 days
    D. 6 months

63. If a record cannot be completed because of the death of a physician, the health information practitioner should
    A. file the incomplete record in the department's permanent file section
    B. forward the record to the facility's medical staff president for completion
    C. refer the incomplete record to the health record committee for action
    D. request that the physician who took over the practice complete the record

64. Pathology (tissue) reports must be completed on
    A. diseased tissue only that is removed at surgery
    B. all tissue removed during a surgical procedure
    C. cancer tissue only or tissue that might be cancerous
    D. tissue sent to the pathologist at the discretion of the surgeon

65. A question on the documentation practices of a particular physician arises through health information department analysis. The health information practitioner should first notify the
    A. chief of the medical staff
    B. hospital administrator
    C. physician in question
    D. health record committee

66. When documenting SOAP notes, reference is made to the problem list by
    A. recording the number and title of the appropriate problem prior to recording the SOAP note
    B. soaping the progress note in that particular section of the patient's health record
    C. duplicating the problem list so that it is filed ahead of the referenced SOAP note
    D. documenting the problem letter and its title before the note is written in the record

67. Which problem-oriented record portion incorporates the history and physical?
    A. problem list
    B. database
    C. SOAP note
    D. initial plans

68. Veterans Health Administration facilities consistently use which of the following as a basis for their numbering system?
    A. social security number as unit number
    B. family numbering for all outpatients
    C. serial-unit numbering and filing system
    D. straight numeric filing and numbering

69. A family numbering system is most useful in
    A. children's hospitals
    B. neighborhood health centers
    C. rehabilitation hospitals
    D. proprietary hospitals

70. The middle digit number filed last in the following series is
    A. 97-26-52
    B. 96-27-51
    C. 95-27-52
    D. 96-27-50

71. With which filing system is quality control most difficult?
    A. unit
    B. middle digit
    C. straight numeric
    D. serial-unit

72. For records of medium thickness, a file guide should be provided for every
    A. 25 records
    B. 50 records
    C. 100 records
    D. 200 records

73. File guides are more permanent with which filing system?
    A. straight numeric
    B. terminal digit
    C. middle digit
    D. serial-unit

74. The more information abstracted into a disease and operation index, the
    A. less time spent retrieving appropriate records
    B. more time spent retrieving appropriate records
    C. less cost in preparing and utilizing the index
    D. less time spent in preparing the indices

75. A terminal digit file guide is labeled: $\frac{40}{30}$. The 40 is considered
    A. primary
    B. secondary
    C. tertiary
    D. terminal

76. A final note serves as a discharge summary in minor cases requiring less than
    A. 24 hours of hospitalization
    B. 36 hours of hospitalization
    C. 48 hours of hospitalization
    D. 72 hours of hospitalization

77. Dr. Dawson performs an operation on a patient and realizes that there is a backlog in transcription turnaround time of operative reports. According to the JCAHO standards, he should
    A. document a comprehensive progress note following surgery
    B. dictate the operative report
    C. wait until the transcription department catches up before he dictates
    D. notify the HIM supervisor regarding the transcription delay

78. As HIM Director, you have been asked to report the incomplete record rate for the month of October at the medical staff meeting. There were 2,250 discharges and 200 incomplete records in the month of October. What would the incomplete record rate be?
    A. .08%
    B. 11%
    C. 8.8%
    D. .11%

79. According to JCAHO requirements, a Type 1 recommendation may be given if the total number of health records delinquent exceeds what percentage of the average monthly discharges?
    A. 25%
    B. 50%

C. 75%
D. 100%

80. All of the following are types of cancer registries EXCEPT:
    A. procedure registry
    B. population based cancer registry
    C. hospital cancer registry
    D. special-purpose registry

81. The chronological listing of all patients in a cancer/tumor registry is called the
    A. tumor registry
    B. accession registry
    C. case finding
    D. case eligibility data

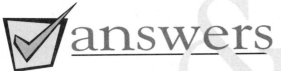

answers & rationales

1.

D. In 1913, the American College of Surgeons (ACS) was founded. In its attempts to raise the standards of surgery, the ACS created a hospital standardization program a few years later. Included in the standards were requirements for complete and accurate health records for all patients. Later, this standardization program was replaced by the organization now known as the Joint Commission on Accreditation of Healthcare Organizations (Abdelhak, pp. 8–9; Johns, pp. 248, 485).

2.

C. The physician may use a rubber stamp under written agreement by the facility that he/she will be the only one using it (Abdelhak, p. 440).

3.

C. All progress notes, reports, test results, etc., are placed in the health record in strict chronological date order, one after the other, no matter the source of each document (Johns, p. 39).

4.

B. Although the health information management department may advise the medical staff in establishing rules and regulations for completion of health records, the development of these regulations is the responsibility of the medical staff. Such regulations should be included in the medical staff's rules and regulations, usually appended to the medical staff bylaws (Abdelhak, pp. 100–101; Johns, p. 490).

5.

C. Secondary medical information includes indexes, registers, logs, etc., that are derived from primary medical information, that is, the health record, and that are individually identifiable by the patient or provider. The emergency room record is a primary source of medical information (Abdelhak, p. 693; Johns, pp. 136, 145–146).

6.

D. The health record is used as a personal document when the identity of the patient is retained and is necessary, which would occur in a malpractice case but not in studies, reports based on grouped data, or surveys conducted by accrediting agencies. Use of the record in these cases would be considered impersonal, because the identity of the patient is not retained (Johns, pp. 138–139).

7.

A. The person writing the error should also sign the correction (Abdelhak, p. 103).

8.

A. All deaths require a discharge summary. A final progress note can be substituted for a discharge summary in the case of patients who are hospitalized less than 48 hours with problems of a minor nature, normal newborns, and uncomplicated obstetrical deliveries. Answers B and C represent complicated cases (Abdelhak, p. 94).

9.

A. A final chart check ensures that all deficiencies have been completed and the record is ready for permanent filing (Abdelhak, pp. 100–101; Johns, pp. 771–777).

10.

D. A summary of the radiation therapy treatment provided is signed by the radiologist and becomes part of the health record (Abdelhak, p. 70; Johns, p. 258).

11.

B. The post anesthesia note can be recorded in the progress notes, recovery room record, or anesthesia report and documents the patient's condition after anesthesia (e.g., nature and extent of anesthesia-related complications). It is documented and signed within 24 hours after surgery by the practitioner who administered the anesthetic (Abdelhak, pp. 95–96; Glondys, p. 146).

12.

B. One of the disadvantages of POMR is that it requires more documentation than other systems; thus, it is not readily accepted by those whose documentation load is already heavy (Abdelhak, pp. 98–99; Johns, pp. 88–89).

13.

D. If a card index becomes too large, inactive cards can be microfilmed. A computerized MPI, of course, solves any space problems inherent with cards (Abdelhak, pp. 189–190; Johns, p. 206).

14.

D. If an initial is given instead of a patient's first or middle name, "file nothing before something." Thus, the sequence for this question is D, A, C, B (Abdelhak, pp. 182–183; Johns, p. 783).

15.

B. Divorce often causes changes in heads of households and in the children who belong to each household. Marriage of children may also change head of household status. These changes make renumbering, refiling, and cross-referencing necessary and are the major disadvantages of family numbering (Abdelhak, pp. 179–180; Johns, pp. 783–784).

16.

B. With serial-unit numbering, inactive records are those remaining at the beginning of the file area, since records of patients readmitted to the facility have been retrieved and incorporated into the newer record further along in the files. Another numbering system that would be easy to purge is serial numbering, because records for inactive storage would be housed at the beginning of the file, as those with the lowest numbers are also the oldest records. With unit numbering, each file must be inspected to determine the last year of treatment. This is a major disadvantage of unit numbering. The type of filing system used (e.g., terminal digit and straight numeric) is irrelevant when considering the ease of purging files (Abdelhak, pp. 179–180; Johns, pp. 769–770).

17.

A. The requisition slip is used to document a request for a record and is usually a multipart form; one copy of the slip is attached to the record for delivery to the requestor; another copy is placed in the outguide, which replaces the record in the file; the third slip is utilized in the department's locator file and arranged in numerical order according to patient number (when the record is returned, this slip and that contained in the outguide are removed and destroyed) (Abdelhak, pp. 194–196; Johns, p. 788).

18.

A. The clue to answering this question is in the phrase, "within a primary section"; the only correct response is A. The other answers represent multiple primary sections of terminal digit files because the primary numbers are the last two digits (Abdelhak, pp. 179–180).

19.

B. Inactive records are not necessarily destroyed; usually they are stored away from the active area (in another area of the facility, off-site, or perhaps on microfilm or optical disk); therefore, the statute of limitations is not an issue in determining inactive status. The chief criterion for determining record inactivity is the amount of space available (Abdelhak, pp. 184, 192; Johns, pp. 205–208).

20.

A. The total number of guides needed for the terminal digit file area has been determined (in this case, 2,000). The student must remember that there are 100 primary sections in a terminal digit file system (from 00 to 99). Divide the 2,000 guides by the 100 primary sections and it is determined that 20 guides are needed within each primary section. Therefore, the pattern on the guides would be every 500 numbers (as seen in answer A) (Abdelhak, pp. 184, 186; Johns, pp. 787–788).

21.

A. In the problem-oriented health record, SOAP notes are the type of progress notes most commonly used, but other notes may also be used, including the common narrative note. Nursing notes are part of the progress notes. The history and physical examination report is part of the database. The initial plan is separate from the other parts of the record (database, problem list, and progress notes/discharge summary) (Abdelhak, pp. 98–99; Johns, p. 39).

22.

A. The admitting department obtains identification and financial data, has the patient or representative sign consent forms, assigns a patient number, and distributes relevant information to various other departments. Sometimes the record begins prior to admission in the form of preadmission testing or other data (NetMBA, p. 1).

23.

A. The review of systems is an interview conducted by the attending physician or representative (e.g., intern in a teaching hospital) that allows the patient to describe subjective symptoms that may help the physician arrive at a diagnosis. Although the format is similar to that used in documenting the physical examination, the information is provided by the patient and is therefore part of the history rather than part of the physical examination (Abdelhak, p. 92).

24.

A. A provisional (tentative) diagnosis is based on information in the history and physical examination. The principal diagnosis is that established after study and the primary diagnosis consumes the most resources during the hospitalization. The chief complaint would be found on the history and is in the patient's own words (Abdelhak, p. 92).

25.

B. Color-coding of folders helps to prevent health records from being filed incorrectly and makes it easier to spot misfiles. It is most effective with terminal digit and middle digit filing systems, although it can also be used with straight numeric filing (Abdelhak, p. 192).

26.

A. The standards of the JCAHO (and those of the American Osteopathic Association), the regulations of the Conditions of Participation of the U.S. Department of Health and Human Services, and state licensing requirements regarding health records establish goals that hospitals strive to meet with regard to the content of health records. Memoranda of Understanding are agreements between hospitals and PROs (Abdelhak, p. 545; Glondys, p. 3; Johns, pp. 829–835).

27.

C. Progress notes include an admission note, follow-up progress notes, and a final note. The final note is the discharge note. In addition, progress notes are documented as the patient's condition warrants and in accordance with medical staff rules and regulations (Abdelhak, pp. 93–93; Glondys, p. 63; Johns, pp. 56–57).

28.

A. Quantitative analysis also includes a review for documentation errors such as missing dates, errors in the proper correction of documentation, and skipped spaces on reports that should be lined through. Review for potentially compensable events, consistency in recording of provider entries, and evaluation of use of abbreviations on the face sheet are features of qualitative analysis (Abdelhak, pp. 100–103; Johns, pp. 204, 776, 777).

29.

B. The newborn is an individual in his or her own right, and as such, has his or her own record generated. The healthy newborn has relatively few forms documented in the record (including admission/discharge form, birth history form, newborn identification form, newborn physical examination, and nursing record). If a newborn is premature or is born with anomalies, the record is expanded to include additional reports as well as specialized forms to document detailed observations (Abdelhak, pp. 90, 96).

30.

C. Incident reports document events that are not consistent with the routine care of a particular patient; these might be adverse patient occurrences or violations of policies and procedures. Once completed, the incident report is filed separately from the patient's record; it serves as an administrative tool (i.e., for the purpose of early detection of problems or potentially compensable events, the incident report serves as a mechanism for the early investigation of serious incidents). While the incident is documented in the record, no mention is made that an incident report was filed. Because the incident report is an administrative tool, it is not subject to disclosure in a lawsuit; should the incident report be referenced in the patient's record, it could become subject to disclosure (Abdelhak, pp. 410, 462; Johns, pp. 502–503).

31.

C. Straight numeric filing involves filing records in exact chronological order according to the patient number (Abdelhak, p. 183; Johns, p. 784).

32.

A. Answers C and D are disadvantages of straight numeric filing. Misfiles are common in straight numeric filing. It is not possible to assign a file section to a particular employee (if more than one employee has the position of file clerk) because all of the file clerks will be filing the most recently discharged health records in the same location. The answer that addresses confidentiality of the health record is irrelevant because the fact that a record is filed by any numbering system rather than patient name allows for a measure of confidentiality (Abdelhak, pp. 182–183; Johns, pp. 769–770).

33.

C. In terminal digit filing, the last two digits are primary, the middle two are secondary, and the first two are tertiary. Therefore, the order of this series of terminal digit numbers would be C, D, A, B (Abdelhak, pp. 184–185; Johns, pp. 784–785).

34.

C. The patient register provides a record of all patient admissions to the facility in chronological order as patients were admitted (Johns, pp. 767–769).

35.

B. There are numerous microforms available, including those mentioned in the question and ultra fiche and computer output microfilm. Each type has distinct advantages, disadvantages, and features (e.g., storage density vs. ability to update microfilm, etc.) (Abdelhak, pp. 206–208; Johns, pp. 786–787).

36.

C. Follow-up on cancer patients is offered for the patient's lifetime to monitor the patient's status. The cancer registry must be persistent in its search for missing information about cancer patients in order to achieve a 90% follow-up rate, the requirement for American College of Surgeons' accreditation of the facility's cancer registry (Abdelhak, p. 274; Johns, pp. 142–143).

37.

D. Bar codes can be preprinted on file folders and used for record tracking in conjunction with a computer software package especially designed for this function. Preprinting the bar codes reduces the risk of potential error as compared with affixing the bar code labels onto file folders as records are used (Abdelhak, pp. 196–198).

38.

A. Birth and death certificates should be kept permanently because copies of them may be requested many years later. If the certificates are contained within the health record, they will automatically be maintained as long as needed (Abdelhak, p. 91; Johns, p. 71).

39.

C. The chief complaint is the reason given by the patient for his or her request for medical care (Abdelhak, p. 86).

40.

D. The hospital provides ancillary services when a patient receives services from a department such as the hospital clinical laboratory or radiology department (Abdelhak, pp. 20–21).

41.

B. A palpable axillary node can be felt (palpated) by the physician. Answer A is a symptom that would be described by a patient during the review of systems done while the history is being taken, or it might be the patient's chief complaint. Answer C would be documented in the patient's past history and answer D is part of the review of systems, which are both documented in the patient's history (Abdelhak, pp. 92–93).

42.

B. Once the purpose of the form is clearly understood, other appropriate decisions (such as answers A, C, and D) about its design can be made (Abdelhak, pp. 159–160; Johns, pp. 778–780).

43.

C. Vital signs are documented in the general survey portion of the physical examination report (Abdelhak, pp. 92–93).

44.

C. The physical examination documents a general survey, which includes the doctor's observations about the height and weight of the patient, the patient's facial expressions, etc. Answers A, B, and D are documented in the physical examination, while answer C is documented in the history report (Abdelhak, pp. 92–93).

45.

A. Standing orders are also called routine orders and are to be signed by the physician when utilized (Abdelhak, p. 93; Johns, p. 52).

46.

C. Analysis of records for deficiencies is quantitative analysis, and would identify the records that needed to be completed by the health care provider. In addition, it would be possible to determine the number of records considered incomplete as well as delinquent, as long as the medical staff had specified a time frame for completion of health records (Abdelhak, pp. 100–103; Johns, pp. 776–777).

47.

B. Each time a patient receives treatment in the facility's emergency department, the JCAHO requires that a record be generated (Abdelhak, pp. 110–111).

48.

A. The POR (or POMR) allows record documentation to be generated in a logical format, starting with the database and continuing by documenting the problem list, initial plans, and progress notes in SOAP format (Abdelhak, pp. 98–99; Johns, pp. 39, 89).

49.

B. Plan statements are documented under the *P* portion of the SOAP note in the problem-oriented record (Abdelhak, pp. 98–99; Johns, pp. 39, 89).

50.

B. The unit numbering system allows for a patient to be assigned a number on the first admission to the hospital, and to retain that same number on subsequent admissions. In this example, several patients were assigned a number for the first time as demonstrated by numbers assigned in the 9000 series; however, three patients were obviously readmissions to the facility as demonstrated by the out-of-sequence numbers assigned to them (Abdelhak, p. 179).

51.

D. When utilizing the social security number as the unit patient number, if a patient does not have a social security number, a pseudonumber may be assigned. The Veterans Health Administration issues pseudonumbers based on designations for the patient's initials for the first three digits and use of the date of birth for the remaining digits (Abdelhak, p. 81; Johns, pp. 127–128).

52.

C. Rotary is a type of microfilm camera (Abdelhak, pp. 209–211; Johns, pp. 786–787).

53.

A. The disease index is arranged according to the code numbers assigned by health information management department personnel, based on the classification system used by the facility (Abdelhak, p. 236; Johns, p. 140).

54.

A. While the annual reports are kept permanently, monthly analyses can be destroyed after 5 years and the daily analyses of hospital services can be destroyed after 2 years (Huffman, p. 308).

55.

D. Other rules for alphabetical filing are provided in Abdelhak, pp. 182–183.

56.

B. The outpatient department utilizes a unit numbering system; therefore, Mary Jones retains the same number she was previously assigned on an outpatient basis (Abdelhak, p. 179; Johns, p. 770).

57.

D. Terminal digit filing has nothing to do with number assignment because all new numbers would be assigned in straight numerical order by the admission department and logged in the number index. With unit numbering, a new patient to the facility would be assigned the most recent patient number available for assignment, in this case response D (Abdelhak, p. 179; Johns, p. 770).

58.

C. The number of incomplete records for the month is 1,763 minus 521, or 1,242. Dividing this number by the total discharges and multiplying by 100 gives the incomplete record rate of 70.45%. Remember the generic formula for rates: The number of times something did happen divided by the number of times something could have happened, multiplied by 100 (Abdelhak, p. 309; Johns, p. 419).

59.

B. The source-oriented record on the nursing unit is organized so that the most current forms within each section are filed on top. The reason is that those persons using the record while the patient is still in the hospital are most concerned with the current status of the patient. After discharge, the record is usually rearranged into chronological date order by section (Abdelhak, p. 98).

60.

A. The number index is a chronological list of the patient identification numbers issued to patients and the name of the patient assigned to each number. The number index helps prevent duplication of numbering or skipped numbers, especially if unit numbering is used (Abdelhak, p. 236).

61.

A. Movable open shelving units on tracks allow the most paper records to be stored in a given amount of space (Abdelhak, pp. 180–181; Johns, p. 785).

62.

C. The provisional autopsy diagnosis is required to be documented within 3 days. The pathologist signs the autopsy report (Abdelhak, p. 95).

63.

C. The health record committee handles issues related to analysis of health records for documentation deficiencies (Abdelhak, p. 104).

64.

B. All tissue removed at surgery must be examined by the pathologist and a report of the findings made. A report must also be made of tissue expelled, biopsies, and autopsies. The pathologist must sign the report (Abdelhak, p. 95; Glondys, p. 147).

65.

C. If only one or two records are involved, the problem may be solved by discussing it with the physician and explaining the consequences. The other answers listed in the question are sources of assistance when the poor documentation practice is widespread, when it deals with quality of care, or when the problem cannot be resolved by working with the individual physician. The nature of the problem governs to whom the problem should be referred if direct communication is ineffective (Abdelhak, p. 100).

66.

A. When the problem list is initially generated, each problem is assigned a number that is referenced each time a SOAP note is written for a particular problem. A separate SOAP note is documented for each problem the practitioner addresses (Abdelhak, p. 99).

67.

B. The database includes the patient's chief complaint, present illness, social data, past history and review of systems, physical examination, and baseline laboratory data (Abdelhak, pp. 98–99; Johns, p. 39).

68.

A. Veterans Health Administration facilities effectively utilize the social security number as the unit number because they receive assistance from the Social Security Administration when determining unknown numbers (Abdelhak, p. 23).

69.

B. With family numbering, one number is assigned to each family, and a pair of digits is placed before this family number to indicate each member of the household in order to differentiate among members of the family. This system is use for neighborhood health centers and mental health centers utilizing family counseling (Abdelhak, pp. 280–281).

70.

B. In middle digit filing, the middle two digits are primary, the first two are secondary, and the last two are tertiary. The correct sequence for filing purposes would be A, C, D, B (Abdelhak, p. 185; Johns, pp. 782–784).

71.

C. The file clerk has to consider all digits of a patient number when filing according to the straight numeric filing system; this increases the chance for misfiles. In addition, because the majority of new records to be filed will be located in the same area of the files, it is not feasible to assign each file clerk responsibility for a specific section of the files (Abdelhak, p. 183; Johns, p. 784).

72.

B. If records are normally quite thick, more frequent file guides should be provided. However, for records of medium thickness, it would be acceptable to place a guide for every 50 records (Abdelhak, pp. 183–184; Johns, pp. 786–788).

73.

B. With straight numeric and middle digit filing, guides have to be added or changed because as new numbers are issued in chronological order, new guides must be placed in the files to reflect numerical increases in the two left-hand digits of the number. In addition, as old records are purged, guides in the affected sections of the file must be changed. In terminal digit filing, guides remain unchanged because primary and secondary digits keep recurring as new patient numbers are assigned. Answer D (serial-unit) is a numbering system (Abdelhak, pp. 183–184; Johns, pp. 786–788).

74.

A. However, the more information abstracted, the higher the cost (Abdelhak, pp. 236, 267).

75.

B. When two pairs of numbers appear on a file guide, the top number is secondary and the bottom number is primary (Abdelhak, pp. 184–185; Johns, pp. 784–785).

76.

C. Final progress notes are appropriate for patients hospitalized for less than 48 hours for minor conditions. If a patient develops complications or dies during hospitalization, a discharge summary must be documented, even though the stay was less than 48 hours. Final progress notes are also acceptable for normal newborns and uncomplicated obstetrical deliveries (Abdelhak, pp. 93–94; Johns, p. 831).

77.

A. According to the Conditions of Participation, "When the operative report is not placed in the health record immediately after surgery, a progress note is entered immediately" (IM.7.3.2.2.2) (Glondys, p. 128).

78.

A. To calculate the incomplete record rate: # incomplete records for given period ÷ # discharges for given period × 100, 200 ÷ 2250 × 100 = 8.8% (Abdelhak, p. 100).

79.

B. According to JCAHO, A Type 1 recommendation may be given if "the number of delinquent records is greater than 50% of the average number of discharged patients per quarter, over the previous 12 months" (Abdelhak, p. 100).

80.

A. Hospital based, population based or central registries, and special-purpose registries are all types of cancer registries. The procedure registry is a fabricated answer (Abdelhak, pp. 264–283; Johns, pp. 141–143).

81.

B. The accession registry is a chronological listing of all cancer patients treated, which is used to assess the annual caseload. The master file is only an alphabetical listing of all patients and does not provide yearly caseload analysis. Case finding is also known as case identification, which means identifying any reportable case of cancer. Case eligibility data is a list that includes the types of cases that are to be included and excluded in the database (Abdelhak pp. 266, 274; Johns, pp. 141–143).

2 Health Care Delivery Systems

objectives

After completion of this chapter, the student will be able to:

➤ Discuss the historical development of health care organizations.

➤ Describe the different regulatory agencies and organizations in health care.

➤ Distinguish between the various health care organizations available.

➤ Differentiate between accreditation, licensure, and legislation in health care.

➤ Discuss the health care team and their respective roles in the health care process.

➤ Outline the organizational structure of the professional staff in health care organizations.

DIRECTIONS (Questions 1–58): Each of the questions or incomplete statements below is followed by suggested answers or completions. Select the **best** answer in each case.

1. Which is responsible for coordinating all hospital clinical activities?
   A. Hospital administration
   B. Executive Committee
   C. Nursing staff
   D. JCAHO

2. Which allows family members who normally provide care to a person to take a break from providing that care?
   A. community care
   B. respite care
   C. rehab care
   D. hospice care

3. Which is a distinctive feature of health maintenance organizations (HMOs)?
   A. There is utilization of a fee-for-service system
   B. Fixed premiums are prepaid for health services
   C. Their mission is to bring health care to the indigent
   D. Seven days per week, 12–16 hours per day care is provided

4. All of the following are considered long-term care facilities EXCEPT:
   A. assisted living facility
   B. substance abuse facility
   C. independent living facility
   D. domiciliary facility

5. Part of the accreditation survey process is listed below in responses A to E. Identify the first step that is out of order.
   A. The interested facility must submit an application and complete a questionnaire
   B. An on-site survey is conducted; the team consists of health care professionals
   C. Surveyors conduct a summation conference with representatives of the facility
   D. The surveyors file their findings in a written report to the accreditation agency
   E. Representatives of the facility have an opportunity to comment on adverse findings

6. A physician who has newly relocated to the area applied and was accepted as an active staff member at the local hospital. The physician will
   A. apply for reappointment and/or renewal of privileges within 2 years
   B. be exempt from serving on medical staff committees for 2 years
   C. work under the direct supervision of another active staff member
   D. report directly to the hospital administrator of the health care facility

DIRECTIONS: Questions 7–10: Match the appropriate type of ambulatory care service with the case scenario.

   A. Ambulatory surgery
   B. Ancillary services
   C. Emergency department
   D. Outpatient department

7. Mrs. Hughston is transported to the hospital after complaining of severe right lower quadrant pain. She is evaluated and undergoes laboratory tests, which prove to be negative. She is discharged to be seen by her primary care physician in his office.

8. Sally Sims is seen in the hospital and undergoes a bilateral mammogram because this type of radiographic equipment is not available in her physician's office.

9. Henry Franklin undergoes a right inguinal herniorrhaphy at 7:00 A.M. and is discharged at noon to return home in order to recuperate.

10. Mary Forbes is registered for her weekly physical therapy and undergoes treatment consisting of whirlpool baths and diathermy.

11. A satellite ambulatory care unit
    A. may or may not be associated with a hospital
    B. is physically separate from the hospital
    C. can be attached to the hospital itself
    D. provides comprehensive care for patients

12. Which statement is characteristic of a group practice?
    A. It consists of a single specialty or multi-specialty and provides comprehensive care
    B. It has management responsibility for providing comprehensive prepaid patient care
    C. It is an organized outpatient department physically separate from the hospital
    D. It is a freestanding facility that provides surgical services only to the patients

13. Mary Jones sustained a laceration to her hand while on the job and was seen in the factory's clinic where the hand was evaluated by the nurse. Ms. Jones was sent to the hospital's emergency department for suturing. This visit to the factory's clinic is a form of
    A. freestanding ambulatory care
    B. hospital outpatient care
    C. on-site ambulatory care
    D. satellite ambulatory care

14. Which is the name of the data set developed by the DHHS and approved by the National Committee on Vital and Health Statistics?
    A. ASTM E1384
    B. UACDS

C. UCDS
D. UHDDS

15. Hospice patients spend the majority of their hospice stay at home. As a result,
    A. many patients receive home care services as part of hospice care
    B. a family member is required to be the primary care person in the home
    C. curative care can be provided to the patient in a convenient manner
    D. it is difficult to arrange for inpatient services when they are deemed necessary

16. All of the following are physicians EXCEPT:
    A. ophthalmologists
    B. osteopaths
    C. anesthesiologists
    D. optometrists

17. CARF accredits
    A. home health agencies
    B. respite care programs
    C. neighborhood health centers
    D. rehabilitation facilities

18. An ambulatory care encounter is defined as
    A. the patient's visit to the facility's outpatient department
    B. a specific identifiable act of service provided to a patient
    C. direct contact between a patient and a health care provider
    D. the course of care a patient receives for a medical problem

19. A nongovernment-owned hospital can be sponsored by any of the following EXCEPT:
    A. municipalities
    B. churches
    C. corporations
    D. individuals

20. Peer Review Organizations obtain government contracts to evaluate the necessity and quality of health services rendered to Medicare patients. Reviews are conducted and judgments are based primarily on the
    A. contract negotiated between patient and Medicare
    B. itemized bill submitted by the health care facility
    C. health care facility's quality management reports
    D. documentation contained within the health record

21. Which is an example of a medical staff rule and regulation?
    A. descriptive policy of medical staff organization
    B. practice of electing medical staff officers
    C. written plan for internal disaster coverage
    D. procedure for amending record documentation

DIRECTIONS: Questions 22–25 refer to the following case study. Mary Jones is recovering from carpal tunnel corrective surgery and received the following services during her October 15 outpatient visit at Anytown Medical Center: urinalysis and hemogram conducted by a lab technician, chest x-ray performed by an x-ray technician, and an initial occupational therapy assessment performed by the facility's occupational therapist. The patient returned to the outpatient department on October 18 and received additional occupational therapy, and then again on October 21, at which time the therapy concluded.

---

22. Calculate the total number of outpatient visits.
    A. one
    B. two
    C. three

D. four
E. five

23. Calculate the total number of encounters occurring between October 15 and 24.
    A. one
    B. two
    C. three
    D. four
    E. five

24. Calculate the total occasions of service occurring between October 15 and 24.
    A. one
    B. two
    C. three
    D. four
    E. five

25. On January 15, the patient underwent an intravenous pyelogram performed by the x-ray technician and interpreted by the radiologist, who also met with the patient briefly; urinalysis performed by the lab technician and interpreted by the pathologist; and one hour of gait training was conducted by the physical therapist in the Physical Therapy Department. How many occasions of service were provided?
    A. one
    B. two
    C. three
    D. four
    E. five

26. Which statement below represents a current trend in the provision of ambulatory care?
    A. ambulatory health care costs will continue to increase dramatically
    B. access to ambulatory health care services will be limited geographically

C. ambulatory health care is being selected as an alternate form of care

D. technological breakthroughs will limit ambulatory health care services

27. Which health maintenance organization model requires employed physicians to treat patients in the organization's facilities?
    A. closed
    B. group
    C. practice
    D. staff

28. The term *nursing facility* is being applied to facilities participating in the Medicaid program and replaces the term
    A. custodial care facility
    B. intermediate care facility
    C. long-term care facility
    D. skilled care facility

29. Compliance by a long-term care facility with which of the following would be considered voluntary?
    A. JCAHO
    B. COP
    C. DOH
    D. OBRA

30. Utilization review of hospice services uses objective criteria to monitor concerns. Review each statement below and select the one that would be considered utilization review monitoring.
    A. routine collection of information pertaining to interdisciplinary team services
    B. identification of problems regarding care delivery to a hospice patient population
    C. documentation of quality assurance program findings resulting in action taken
    D. evaluation of appropriateness of level of hospice and team services provided

31. A physician who is an active member in one hospital and applies to admit an occasional patient to another is applying for what kind of medical staff membership at the second facility?
    A. active
    B. consulting
    C. courtesy
    D. honorary

32. A multidisciplinary team approach in mental health care allows for participation in monitoring and documenting the patient's progress during and response to treatment. Which documentation system would best allow for the above process?
    A. integrated record
    B. patient management
    C. problem-oriented
    D. source-oriented

33. A health care facility receives notification from the Joint Commission on Accreditation of Healthcare Organizations that it has received an accreditation with commendation. This means that
    A. the facility was in almost total compliance with the JCAHO standards
    B. within an 18-month time frame the facility will undergo self-assessment
    C. a plan of correction must be completed by the facility within 6 months
    D. reaccreditation will be unnecessary in the future as it is automatically renewable

34. Which gives legal approval for a facility to offer services?
    A. accreditation
    B. certification
    C. licensure
    D. regulation

35. Upon review of discharged health records, the analysis clerk notices that one physician is consistent in his lack of timely discharge summary documentation. He has previously been notified of this problem. Next, the analysis clerk should
    A. speak directly to the physician responsible
    B. notify the health record committee of the findings
    C. bring the situation to the attention of administration
    D. talk with her supervisor about the situation

36. Revisions of report forms created for use in the record must be approved by the
    A. hospital administrator
    B. HIM committee
    C. health information manager
    D. state department of health

37. A factory guaranteed that all employees would seek care at the local hospital and was able to negotiate a special reduced rate for care rendered. This is a (an)
    A. health maintenance organization
    B. independent practice association
    C. point-of-service plan
    D. preferred provider organization

38. Which form would provide the basic facts about a long-term care resident who has been transferred from a hospital?
    A. admission assessment
    B. admitting evaluation
    C. comprehensive care plan
    D. referral statement

39. An accident report was generated on Joe Poole when he was found on the floor next to his nursing facility bed. Mr. Poole was evaluated and found to be unharmed by the presumed fall. The staff responsible for caring for Mr. Poole completed an accident report and
    A. filed it in the clinical record and documented a progress note about the resident's fall
    B. forwarded it to the nursing facility administrator's executive office for safekeeping
    C. gave it to the patient's family for use in any possible litigation regarding the fall
    D. documented a clinical record progress note and forwarded the report to the CEO

40. The release of health records that contain information about a drug addiction for which the patient sought treatment is controlled by
    A. federal regulation
    B. JCAHO
    C. Medicare COP
    D. state statutes

41. A minimum data set is mandated for use in certified long-term care facilities. The federal requirements that address this document are found under
    A. Medicare COP
    B. CFR 483.20
    C. PL 94-63
    D. ASTM E1384

42. The increase in home health care services being offered has resulted in a (an)
    A. decrease in acute care facility lengths of stay
    B. decrease in number of home health patients
    C. increase in the country's costs of health care
    D. increase in long-term care facility admissions

43. A home health care aide bathes a patient in her home on March 15. A nurse sees the pa-

tient on that day to administer an insulin injection. On March 16, the aide returns to bathe the patient; the nurse returns to administer another insulin injection. How many visits will the agency be allowed to bill Medicare?

A. one

B. two

C. three

D. four

44. The JCAHO requires mental health care facilities to conduct several types of quality assurance reviews. Review the list below and select the type of review that would be more characteristic of that conducted in a mental health care facility than a hospital.

A. review of medication errors

B. review of experimental drugs

C. review of adverse effects

D. review of drug records

45. Which has ultimate authority and responsibility for providing proper care to hospital patients?

A. governing board

B. hospital administrator

C. medical staff

D. nursing staff

46. Sally Smith underwent emergency surgery in the hospital's day surgery unit and stayed a total of 18 hours. The care rendered during this time was

A. ambulatory care

B. ancillary care

C. emergency care

D. inpatient care

47. Programs designed to bring health care to the economically disadvantaged are called

A. convenience care centers

B. on-site ambulatory care centers

C. neighborhood health centers

D. preferred provider centers

48. A facility that has a medical staff consisting of MDs and DOs desires American Osteopathic Association accreditation status. It is also currently accredited by the Joint Commission on Accreditation of Healthcare Organizations. This facility

A. must use the term *osteopathic* in the facility's title and on its stationery

B. is mandated by federal law to ask permission of the JCAHO before proceeding

C. will find that the AOA accreditation process is similar to that of the JCAHO

D. can expect to be granted up to a 5-year accreditation status by the AOA

49. A local hospital expanded its services offered to the community and operates an urgent care center across town in addition to the hospital. This would now be considered a

A. multihospital system

B. single hospital ownership

C. corporation-owned facility

D. voluntary community facility

50. A departmentalized medical staff is organized according to service. What is the title of the individual who is responsible for directing the functions of each service?

A. chairperson

B. supervisor

C. coordinator

D. administrator

51. Medicare would categorize a county health department home health agency as

A. provider-based

B. proprietary

C. private nonprofit

D. government

52. The health information manager who investigates the establishment of a policy for mental health record retention should first
    A. meet with the facility's administration to solicit their suggestions
    B. survey clinical staff to determine their needs to review original records
    C. evaluate the amount of space available in the clinical record department
    D. check the state mental health code for record retention requirements

53. Home health care agencies have established a portion of the record that can be maintained in the home. Information contained in this record would include all EXCEPT:
    A. emergency plans
    B. patient instructions
    C. plan of treatment
    D. agency staff names

54. An 85-year-old female home health patient requires assistance with daily bathing, weekly housecleaning, and daily preparation of one meal. She is recovering from recent hip replacement surgery on the right. She has completely recovered from the left hip replacement surgery she underwent 3 months ago. The home health agency reviewed her request and assigned a caregiver. Unfortunately, a home health aide was unavailable for this assignment; the agency sent a nurse to perform the above tasks. This is an example of
    A. cost overutilization
    B. cost underutilization
    C. essential medical care
    D. medical necessity

55. Many long-term care facilities perform chart thinning. This means that
    A. lightweight folders are used for discharged records because chart activity levels will be low in long-term care facilities
    B. only basic information is retained in the permanent long-term care health record after the required retention period
    C. material is removed from the active portion of the record and kept in a central location of the health care facility
    D. patients with multiple admissions to the facility (and multiple charts) have the current record available on the unit

56. Rehabilitative care requires coordination of health disciplines to facilitate a successful patient outcome. A critical factor in the coordination of the rehabilitation process is
    A. case management
    B. discharge planning
    C. establishment of goals
    D. preadmission evaluation

57. Because the clinical record is a confidential document, release of information must be handled in such a way that no unauthorized person has access to the record. Another consideration is the situation in which a patient is transferred from one facility to another. The transferring facility forwards copies of records to the receiving facility; this information from the transferring facility is placed in the receiving facility's health record. Upon discharge of the patient from the second facility, the insurance company responsible for paying for the stay requests copies of any and all records on this particular patient. How should the receiving facility handle the rerelease of copies of the transferring facility's health record?
    A. release only that information generated during patient treatment at the receiving facility; do not rerelease information obtained from previous settings
    B. release the transferring facility's health record as requested after first obtaining

permission from their health information management department

C. release any information requested because the contract established between the transferring and receiving facilities would allow for this

D. release information from the transferring facility's health record after first instructing the insurance company to obtain patient permission to do so

58. Who has primary responsibility for the home health care client's plan of care?

A. a home health care agency nurse who cares for the patient

B. a local hospital that has previously treated the patient

C. the family member responsible for the patient's care at home

D. the patient's attending physician (who sees the patient in the office)

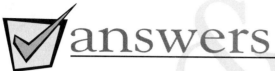

answers & rationales

1.

B. Hospital administration is responsible for establishing an environment in which direct health care services are provided. The nursing staff coordinates the factors that influence the patient's health (e.g., administration of medications, following-through on tests ordered, etc.). The Joint Commission establishes standards for hospitals in the United States and Canada (Abdelhak, p. 28; Johns, pp. 266–267).

2.

B. Respite care might be provided at home or outside of the home, such as in nursing homes and adult day care centers. Hospice programs provide palliative medical care to the terminal patient and psychosocial and spiritual support to the family and patient. Rehabilitative care consists of an extensive range of services provided in many types of rehabilitation facilities. "Community care" is a term fabricated by the authors (Johns, pp. 78–79).

3.

B. Health Maintenance Organizations are defined by the American Hospital Association as "organizations that have management responsibility for providing comprehensive health care services on a prepayment basis to voluntarily enrolled persons within a designated population." Neighborhood health centers attempt to provide care to the economically disadvantaged (i.e., indigent). Preferred provider organizations utilize a fee-for-service system. Urgent care centers are often open 12 to 16 hours/day, 7 days/week (Abdelhak, p. 43).

4.

B. Drug treatment centers consist of settings that are either outpatient, acute, in-patient treatment, or recovery/intervention programs (Peden, p. 226).

5.

D. The representatives of the facility have the opportunity to comment at the conclusion of the summation conference and before the written report is submitted to the accrediting body by the surveyors. In addition, the facility receives a copy of this written report and is permitted to respond in writing regarding the findings (Abdelhak, p. 386; Johns, pp. 485, 775).

6.

A. A is the correct answer. B, C, and D are fabricated responses (Abdelhak, pp. 415–422).

7.

C. According to Abdelhak and colleagues, an emergency patient receives care for conditions that are urgent, life threatening, or potentially disabling. Hospitals see many patients in their emergency departments for a range of problems, such as that listed in this case scenario (Abdelhak, p. 21).

8.

B. This patient was referred by her primary care physician to the hospital's radiology department. The patient is provided with a requisition for ancillary services and a report of services rendered is submitted to the primary care physician. The patient will see this physician in follow-up after the service is rendered (Abdelhak, p. 20).

9.

A. Ambulatory surgery patients do not require an inpatient bed. They typically come to the facility in the early hours of the morning and are discharged later that same day after a period of postoperative observation (Abdelhak, pp. 18–20).

10.

D. This patient received outpatient physical therapy. She would have registered in the outpatient department prior to being seen by the physical therapist (Abdelhak, p. 20).

11.

B. Hospitals may locate a portion of their organized outpatient services physically separate from the main hospital. Satellite ambulatory care units offer primary care, comprehensive care, or services for populations with special needs (Abdelhak, p. 20).

12.

A. A group practice is a facility of three or more physicians and/or dentists who share office space, equipment, office personnel, expenses, etc. A single-specialty practice can consist of several physicians (e.g., a group practice of internal medicine specialists). An HMO provides comprehensive prepaid care to a patient population; satellite ambulatory care units are physically separate from a hospital; and ambulatory surgery facilities provide for outpatient surgery in a hospital (Abdelhak, pp. 18–19; Johns, pp. 357–361).

13.

C. On-site ambulatory care is offered in nonhospital settings such as businesses, educational institutions, and prisons. A freestanding ambulatory care setting includes a physician's office or a neighborhood health center; hospital outpatient care includes the provision of emergency department care, day surgery, and ancillary services; satellite ambulatory care is provided by an organized outpatient department that is physically separate from the hospital (Abdelhak, pp. 18–21; Johns, pp. 276–278, 720).

14.

B. The American Society of Testing and Materials established the ASTM E1384 Standard for the Structure and Content of the Computer-Based Health record and is responsible for vocabulary related to the computer-based health record. The Uniform Clinical Data Set (UCDS) is a national case screening system. The Uniform Hospital Discharge Data Set has been in use for more than 20 years and is the minimum requirement for the collection of Medicare/Medicaid hospital discharge data. The Uniform Ambulatory Care Data Set (UACDS) was approved in 1989 and defines a common core of data collected in ambulatory care settings (Abdelhak, pp. 55, 79, 113, 114).

15.

A. Many hospice organizations establish home health agencies within their realm to care for hospice patients at home; other hospice organizations establish contracts with local home health agencies in order to provide home care for the hospice patient. While a primary care person responsible for looking after the patient in the home is assigned in almost all hospice cases, the individual need not be a relative. The hospice also arranges or contracts for inpatient care with an acute care facility (Abdelhak, pp. 32–33; Johns, pp. 78–79).

16.

D. Optometrists are not physicians (who hold a doctorate in medicine or osteopathy), although they are doctors (of optometry). Ophthalmologists are physicians who specialize in diseases of the eye. Anesthesiologists are physicians who specialize in anesthesiology. Osteopaths obtain a doctor of osteopathy degree from an approved school of osteopathy and become licensed physicians (Abdelhak, p. 28).

17.

D. The Commission on Accreditation of Rehabilitation Facilities provides standards particular to rehabilitation facilities. As with the Joint Commission on Accreditation of Healthcare Organizations, a facility voluntarily undergoes the survey process (Abdelhak, p. 15; Johns, p. 249).

18.

C. Answer A defines a hospital outpatient visit, answer B an occasion of service, and answer D an episode of care (Abdelhak, p. 18).

19.

A. A municipally owned hospital is a city-owned or county-owned hospital and therefore a government-owned facility (Abdelhak, p. 23).

20.

D. PROs review aspects of patient care and they often base their judgments on what is in health records. The contract between the patient and Medicare provides for the review process and the itemized bill from the facility can help identify cases that should be reviewed by the PRO. Quality management reports are considered secondary records and are protected by state law from discovery as legal documents (Abdelhak, pp. 248–249, 451–452; Johns, pp. 28, 31).

21.

D. Rules and regulations outline the mechanisms and details implementing the bylaws. The bylaws define the principles and policies with which medical staff agrees to comply (Abdelhak, pp. 26, 417–419).

22.

C. An outpatient visit is a patient encounter to one or more units or facilities located in or directed by the entity maintaining the outpatient health care services. In this case scenario, the patient had outpatient visits on October 15, 18, and 21; this totals three outpatient visits (Abdelhak, pp. 87, 109).

23.

C. An encounter is the face-to-face contact between a patient and a provider. This patient encountered a provider of care (the occupational therapist) on three occasions. The contacts that the patient had with the laboratory technician and x-ray technician are not considered encounters since these professionals are not considered health care providers (Abdelhak, pp. 17, 20).

24.

(E) An occasion of service is a specific identifiable instance of an act of service involved in the care of patients. This patient received service via the performance of a urinalysis and hemogram in the lab, chest x-ray in the radiology department, and occupational therapy three times; thus, the patient had five occasions of service (Abdelhak, p. 17).

25.

C. An occasion of service is a specific identifiable instance of an act of service involved in the care of patients. This patient received service via the performance of a urinalysis in the lab, IVP in the radiology department, and 1 hour of gait training in the physical therapy department; thus, the patient had three occasions of service (Abdelhak, p. 20).

26.

C. Government control of health care costs continues to influence consumer demand for ambulatory health care services; utilization of alternatives to inpatient care will continue to increase as a result. Comparatively, ambulatory health care costs are lower than inpatient care. Ambulatory care access continues to increase geographically; technological breakthroughs allow more services to be provided in ambulatory care facilities (Abdelhak, pp. 17, 108).

27.

D. Group models (or closed HMOs) contract with physicians who work in their own private offices and usually see only health maintenance organization patients; independent practice associations (IPAs) allow physicians to practice in their own private offices, seeing HMO as well as private-practice patients (Abdelhak, p. 43).

28.

B. Long-term care facility is a term that includes intermediate and skilled care levels provided to patients; skilled care is the most comprehensive level while intermediate care is not as complex. Custodial care is provided to patients in a nursing facility; however, no long-term care facilities are dedicated to providing custodial care because they would not receive reimbursement for patients receiving only this level of care under the Medicaid program (Abdelhak, p. 31).

29.

A. The Joint Commission on Accreditation of Healthcare Organizations develops standards for long-term care facilities; the process of accreditation by the Joint Commission is considered voluntary, unlike the regulatory, mandatory compliance with federal conditions of participation and state department of health licensure laws. OBRA refers to the Omnibus Budget Reconciliation Act passed in 1987 and implemented in 1991; this law changed the focus of long-term care, revising and consolidating requirements for facilities to receive Medicare and Medicaid reimbursement (Abdelhak, p. 58; Johns, p. 248).

30.

D. The first three choices in this question represent quality assurance as conducted in a hospice; answer *D.* refers to utilization review monitoring (Abdelhak, pp. 406–407; Johns, pp. 495–496).

31.

C. A consulting staff member provides consulting services for a specific problem when requested. Honorary members are so designated for outstanding contributions or service; they are often granted this status at retirement from active membership.

Active members render the majority of patient care, hold office, and serve on committees. Those who have applied for active status and have not yet been approved are often granted associate membership (Abdelhak, pp. 415–416).

32.

C. The integrated record involves organizing all reports within the record according to strict chronological date format, regardless of type of report; most facilities modify this process and integrate just progress notes so that all professionals (e.g., physical therapists, physicians, nurses, etc.) document on a common set of progress notes. The problem-oriented record can incorporate the integrated recordkeeping approach; however, the integrated record does not necessarily require implementation of the problem-oriented approach to recordkeeping. The source-oriented record is least favorable because information is scattered throughout the record. Patient management refers to the process utilized in mental health care when admitting a patient for treatment: intake, assessment of the patient, frequency of documentation, progress notes, documentation of discharge summary, and plans for aftercare (Abdelhak, pp. 98–100; Johns, p. 88–90).

33.

A. Although a facility is in almost total compliance with JCAHO standards, the facility will still undergo the full accreditation procedure when the current accreditation status expires. About 18 months after a survey, the facility receives correspondence from the Joint Commission containing a reminder to continue performing self-assessment and to correct any recommendations received in its last survey. A plan of correction must be performed if the facility receives conditional accreditation. In addition, a follow-up survey is performed to determine ultimate accreditation status. No facility is exempt from the reaccreditation process, even if it is in almost total compliance with JCAHO (Abdelhak, p. 58; Johns, p. 248).

34.

C. Accreditation is associated with agencies such as the Joint Commission on Accreditation of Healthcare Organizations. Certification refers to Medicare Certification conducted by the Department of Health and Human Services. An example of regulation is the Conditions of Participation, requirements for facility reimbursement under the Medicare program (Abdelhak, p. 14; Johns, pp. 86–87).

35.

D. If the physician had not been previously notified of this particular deficiency, the analysis clerk could speak directly to the physician. In this case, however, because of the organization structure of the department, it is appropriate for the clerk to take the matter to her supervisor for resolution. The supervisor could take it to the health record committee as an agenda item (administration would become aware of the problem at that time) (Abdelhak, p. 100; Johns, pp. 776–777).

36.

B. Health care facilities have a forms committee or a subcommittee of the health record committee, which approves the design of forms for use in the health record (Johns, pp. 780–781).

37.

D. The HMO provides comprehensive prepaid care to a patient population; an IPA is an example of an HMO; and a point-of-service plan is a form of managed care that utilizes the primary care physician as a gatekeeper of care to be rendered (Abdelhak, pp. 43–44; Johns, pp. 285, 340, 358).

38.

D. The referral statement or "transfer statement" usually accompanies the resident from the hospital to the nursing facility. The admitting evaluation or assessment is performed for each resident upon admission to the nursing facility. The comprehensive care plan is begun when the resident is admitted and provides a working tool with input from each discipline involved in care (Abdelhak, p. 118).

39.

D. The accident report is also called an incident report. It is never filed in the clinical record, but is forwarded to the facility's CEO or risk manager for filing purposes. It is appropriate for the facility staff to document a progress note about the incident; they should not mention that an incident or accident report has been filed (Abdelhak, p. 410; Johns, pp. 502–503).

40.

A. Federal regulation pertaining to the confidentiality of alcohol and drug abuse records are found in Title 42, Part 2 of the Federal Regulations (Abdelhak, pp. 443–444; Johns, p. 70).

41.

B. Medicare Conditions of Participation includes federal regulations that facilities must meet for keeping health records in order to seek reimbursement from Medicare and Medicaid. PL 94-63 (Special Health Revenue Sharing Act of 1975) contains amendments covering numerous items that relate to services offered by mental health care facilities, etc. ASTM E1384 (American Society of Testing and Materials E1384) includes the Standard for the Structure and Content of the Computer-Based Health record (Abdelhak, pp. 55, 128, 704; Motley, p. 1).

42.

A. Cost containment measures (in addition to an increasing population of elderly persons, consumerism, and improved medical technology) have resulted in an increase in the number of home care providers offering services (Johns, p. 278).

43.

D. A visit is every time a health worker furnishes home health services to the beneficiary (Abdelhak, p. 31; Johns, pp. 342–343).

44.

B. The Joint Commission requires that mental health care facilities review all of the answers listed in response to the question. The best choice in answer to this question would be experimental drugs because this type of review would be unique to mental health care as compared with general hospital care (Johns, p. 248).

45.

A. The governing board delegates authority for non-medical activities to the hospital administrator or chief executive officer and for medical activities to the medical staff (Abdelhak, p. 24).

46.

A. Ambulatory surgery provides surgical services to patients who do not require an inpatient bed. Ancillary services consist of laboratory, radiology, etc., provided on an inpatient, emergency, or outpatient basis. Emergency services are provided to patients who need care on an urgent basis. Inpatient services are provided to patients who require overnight admission to the hospital (Abdelhak, p. 18–21).

47.

C. Treatment in neighborhood health centers is typically family centered. The centers seek to reduce barriers to the access of care and to keep costs low. Emphasis is placed on preventive medicine and education. Preferred provider organizations, not centers, offer a benefit package to subscribers that include physician and hospital services, as well as other services. Convenience care centers (or urgent care centers) typically offer 12–16 hours/day, 7 days/week care for routine or minor emergency conditions. On-site ambulatory care is provided in a nonhospital setting such as a company's premises (Abdelhak, p. 19; Johns, p. 285).

48.

C. Facilities that have MD and DO physicians on staff are not required to use the osteopathic designation in the facility title. They can seek both AOA and JCAHO accreditation. Response B is fabricated. The AOA grants 1-, 2-, or 3-year accreditations to hospitals (Abdelhak, pp. 421–422; Johns, p. 490).

49.

B. A multihospital system consists of two or more hospitals that are leased, sponsored, or contract-managed by a central organization. There is not enough information in the example to identify whether the facility is voluntary or proprietary, so those responses are incorrect (Abdelhak, pp. 33–34).

50.

A. The chairperson of a medical staff department (e.g., surgery) is responsible for implementing a process for monitoring and evaluating the quality and appropriateness of patient care rendered as well as the performance of individuals with clinical privileges in the department (Abdelhak, pp. 467–468).

51.

D. CMS defines five major Medicare provider home health agency categories (the four choices given, and also voluntary nonprofit). The government category includes the state or local health and welfare department. The voluntary nonprofit category includes visiting nurse associations; provider-based is also known as hospital-based; proprietary are for-profit providers; and private nonprofit providers are owned privately and have nonprofit status (Abdelhak, p. 31).

52.

D. Checking with the state mental health code is the logical first step; all of the other answers listed as responses would be appropriate as follow-up to checking the mental health code (Johns, pp. 205–207).

53.

C. The plan of treatment is part of the home care health record, housed at the agency's office and not in the patient's home (Abdelhak, pp. 119–120).

54.

A. Cost overutilization occurs "when a caregiver is used beyond the level of medical necessity, such as a registered nurse who is used to bathe and turn a patient." Cost underutilization "occurs when the caregiver is not trained to provide the level of care that is demanded, such as a licensed practical nurse administering chemotherapy." Medical necessity "is the appropriateness and medical necessity for the level of care provided." Essential medical care is a phrase fabricated by the authors (Abdelhak, pp. 402–406; Johns, pp. 255–256).

55.

C. Chart thinning refers to the removal of older information from the long-term care active record; this information is stored remotely from the nursing unit. Lightweight folders are used to house records in a long-term care facility because of the reduced record activity upon discharge or expiration of the patient (as compared with an acute care facility, for example). Long-term care facilities must refer to state and other regulations, federal regulations, accrediting standards, and a review of record usage after discharge to develop a record retention schedule; basic information retained permanently after records are destroyed include resident name, date of birth, and admission and discharge dates. Answer D is fabricated (Abdelhak, pp. 183–184; Johns, pp. 786–788).

56.

B. Discharge planning is crucial to the rehabilitation process because the patient's level of self-sufficiency is established as a physical objective to be realized on a social and environmental level. Case management is an approach utilized by employer-sponsored review programs to coordinate the patient's rehab potential, medical services, and ability to return to an appropriate productive employment situation. Preadmission evaluation is conducted as part of rehabilitation care utilization management. Establishing goals is a necessary part of the assessment process prior to a patient's admission to a rehabilitation program (Abdelhak, p. 98).

57.

A. When information is released from the present facility's record, the only material it is empowered to release is that generated during the course of treatment at the facility. There should be no rerelease of information obtained from previous settings. It is possible that a transferring facility may give permission for the receiving facility to rerelease information from its health record; this would be unusual and should be avoided. Releasing copies of the transferring facility's records is prohibited (Huffman, pp. 192–193, 586).

58.

D. The physician must document the patient's care with a plan of treatment and reviewed at least once every 60 days along with a patient summary forwarded to the patient's attending physician and to the referral source at least every 61 days (Abdelhak, pp. 120–126; Johns, pp. 77–78).

3 Classification Systems

objectives

After completion of this chapter, the student will be able to:

- Distinguish between the various nomenclatures and classification systems.

- Discuss the current coding systems utilized in health care organizations.

- Identify the contents of the CPT-4 coding system.

- Identify the inpatient and outpatient coding principles as outlined in the Official Guidelines for ICD-9-CM Coding.

- Describe the purpose of case-mix classification systems.

- List the different severity of illness systems and the variations.

- Describe encoding systems and advantages and disadvantages of computer-assisted encoders.

- Select the principal diagnosis and principal procedure in a case scenario.

- Select and differentiate between comorbidities and complications in a case scenario.

DIRECTIONS (Questions 1–76): Each of the questions or incomplete statements below is followed by suggested answers or completions. Select the **best** answer in each case.

1. A systematic listing of names used in any science or art is a
   A. classification
   B. nomenclature
   C. dictionary
   D. glossary

2. The instructional term *See* in Volume 2/Alphabetic Index of ICD-9-CM
   A. identifies codes used when information is needed to code to a more specific category
   B. directs the coder to a more specific term under which the correct code can be found
   C. indicates further information is available that may provide an additional diagnosis code
   D. defines terms, clarifies information, or lists choices for additional digits (i.e., fifth digits)

3. NOS is an abbreviation that
   A. provides instruction that a condition is to be coded elsewhere and is associated with the *excludes* notes found in the first volume of the ICD-9-CM manual
   B. identifies codes and terms to be used only when information necessary to code the diagnosis to a more specific category is not found in ICD-9-CM
   C. indicates that the ICD-9-CM code is unspecified and, if possible, the coder should seek additional information so that a more precise code can be assigned
   D. appears under three-digit category codes to further define or give an example of the contents of the category in Volume 1 of the ICD-9-CM manual

4. In Volume 2/Alphabetic Index, the primary arrangement of main terms is by

   A. condition
   B. site
   C. morphology
   D. body system

5. With a differential diagnosis on a discharged inpatient chart (e.g., acute pancreatitis vs. acute cholecystitis; depressive reaction or hypothyroidism), which should be coded?
   A. both diagnoses
   B. neither diagnosis
   C. the principal diagnosis
   D. the primary diagnosis

6. The CPT coding manual is published annually by the
   A. American Hospital Association
   B. American Medical Association
   C. Centers for Medicare & Medicaid Services
   D. American College of Surgeons

7. A partial mastectomy is assigned CPT-4 code 19160. The procedure was performed bilaterally; the modifier for bilateral procedures is −50. The appropriate way to report the procedure for physician reimbursement is
   A. 19160, 19160-50
   B. 19160, 09950
   C. 19160-99, 19160-50
   D. 19160-09950

8. CPT uses a semicolon to save space and make it easier for the coders to select the most appropriate code without reading redundant material. Choose the appropriate interpretation of the code number 31365 from the following codes and descriptions:

   31360 Laryngectomy; total, without radical neck dissection

   31365 total, with radical neck dissection

31367 subtotal supraglottic, without radical neck dissection

A. Total laryngectomy without radical neck dissection

B. Total laryngectomy with/without radical neck dissection

C. Total radical neck dissection with laryngectomy

D. Total laryngectomy with radical neck dissection

9. When an asterisk appears to the right of the code number, it indicates that the package concept does not apply. The coder would assign a code for preoperative services and for the procedure performed. One of the specific rules addressing the use of asterisks in the Surgery Section states, "When the starred procedure is carried out at the time of an initial visit (new patient) and this procedure constitutes the major service at that visit, procedure number 99025 is listed in lieu of the usual initial visit as an additional service."

CASE EXAMPLE: A new patient is seen in the office for incision and drainage of a simple hematoma. The coder identifies the following potential codes to be assigned: 10140* Incision and Drainage of hematoma; simple. 99025 Initial visit when starred surgical procedure constitutes major service at that visit. 99203 Office or other outpatient visit, new patient. Which combination would be coded for the above case example?

    A. 10140

    B. 99025

    C. 10140, 99025

    D. 99203

    E. 10140, 99025, 99203

10. When dealing with services rendered to treat complications associated with procedures, remember that

    A. such treatment is included in the original code number assigned

B. the patient is not treated for complications; thus no code is assigned

C. a code is assigned to each service rendered to treat the complication

D. the patient is referred to a specialist for treatment of the complication

11. The alphabetical index to E codes is contained in

    A. ICD-9-CM, Volume 1

    B. ICD-9-CM, Volume 2

    C. ICD-9-CM, Volume 3

    D. a separate E code volume

12. "Use additional code if desired" is interpreted to mean that

A. the coder assigns additional ICD-9-CM diagnosis codes at his or her discretion

B. the attending physician should be consulted before assigning the additional codes

C. policies should be developed as to whether or not to assign the additional codes

D. the coder must add further information by using an additional code assignment

13. NEC is an abbreviation that

A. communicates to the coder that a condition is to be coded elsewhere; this abbreviation is associated with *includes* notes found in Volume 1

B. identifies codes and terms to be used only when information necessary to code the diagnosis to a more specific category is not found in ICD-9-CM

C. indicates that the ICD-9-CM code is unspecified and, if possible, the coder should seek additional information so that a more precise code can be assigned

D. appears under three-digit category codes to further define or give an example of the contents of the category in Volume 1 of the ICD-9-CM manual

14. Which of the following disease names is an eponym?
    A. Holmes' syndrome
    B. AIDS
    C. Miscarriage
    D. Carcinoma

15. The discharged inpatient diagnostic statement, "rule out diabetes mellitus," should be
    A. coded as a suspected condition
    B. not coded for this patient case
    C. coded if the condition has been ruled out
    D. coded using a V code from ICD-9-CM

16. CPT distinguishes between benign and malignant lesions regarding
    A. excision
    B. repair
    C. grafting
    D. injection

17. Which explain(s) the contents of subsections in CPT-4?
    A. Notes
    B. Introduction
    C. Guidelines
    D. Instructions

18. Descriptions in the CPT-4 index are arranged according to
    A. the specific section of the CPT-4 coding manual
    B. the anatomy of the human body, from head to toe
    C. the physician's specialty (e.g., pathology, surgery, etc.)
    D. the procedure, anatomic site, eponyms, and other indicators

19. If the coder submitted the code 93010 (Electrocardiogram; interpretation and report only) for reimbursement purposes, it would mean that the physician

    A. performed the electrocardiogram, interpreted it, and dictated a report
    B. performed an electrocardiogram tracing, interpreted it, and dictated a report
    C. interpreted and prepared (documented) the patient's electrocardiogram report
    D. performed, interpreted, and prepared a report on the patient's electrocardiogram

20. The triangle used in CPT means that
    A. a second code number is to be assigned
    B. there is a revised CPT code description
    C. there is a new code in this edition of CPT
    D. special rules apply to these CPT codes

21. HCPCS was developed by
    A. CMS
    B. CPT-4
    C. HHS
    D. WHO

22. Parentheses
    A. are used after an incomplete term that needs one or more of the modifiers that follow to make it assignable to a given category within the ICD-9-CM coding manual
    B. enclose a series of terms, each of which is modified by the statement appearing at the right of the punctuation mark(s) in Volume 2 of the ICD-9-CM coding manual
    C. contain supplementary words that may be present or absent in the statement of a disease or procedure, without affecting the code number to which it is assigned
    D. are nonessential modifiers that follow the main term to clarify the diagnoses and must be present in the diagnostic statement in order for the coder to assign the code

23. The term *and* in a title should be interpreted as
    A. including
    B. and/or
    C. also
    D. with

24. In the diagnosis "acute and chronic bronchitis," which would be coded?
    A. acute bronchitis only
    B. chronic bronchitis only
    C. the condition that occurred first
    D. both acute and chronic bronchitis

25. In 2003, CPT code 86681 was deleted from the code book and the coder is instructed to report code 86255, 86256 instead. If the coder uses last year's edition of the code book and submits code 86681, which of the following will occur?
    A. the documentation in the patient's record will be in error
    B. the fiscal intermediary will change the code assignment
    C. the insurance company will require a special report
    D. the provider will not be eligible for pre-calculated payment rates

26. Regarding fractures or dislocations, reduction and manipulation
    A. mean an attempted restoration of the fracture was performed
    B. are performed on patients who have open fractures or dislocations
    C. correlate with the type of fracture sustained by the patient
    D. are terms that do not mean the same thing; they are antonyms

27. The package concept applies to Surgery Section codes and includes, as an example, the service as described, local infiltration, metacarpal/digital block or topical anesthesia, and
    A. surgeon specialization
    B. preoperative evaluation
    C. physical status modifiers
    D. uncomplicated follow-up care

28. It is possible for procedures to be performed as essential parts of whole procedures not listed separately. An obstetrics patient that receives all of her care from one physician would have this service reported using an all-inclusive code. This patient would be assigned code
    A. 59426 antepartum care only; 7 or more visits
    B. 59400-22 total obstetrical care; unusual services
    C. 59400 routine obstetrical care (of the patient)
    D. 59430 postpartum care only (provided to the patient)

29. The surgeon performed a meniscectomy on a patient. Possible CPT-4 code descriptions include
    EXCISION
    27332 Arthrotomy, with excision of semilunar cartilage (meniscectomy) knee; medial OR lateral
    ARTHROSCOPY
    29881 Arthroscopy, knee, surgical; with meniscectomy (medial OR lateral, including any meniscal shaving)
    Which would cause the description of the procedure to be listed under the above separate headings?
    A. presence of semicolons
    B. use of parentheses
    C. surgical approach
    D. anatomical site

30. ICD-9-CM, Volume 1, contains
    A. tabular list of V codes
    B. alphabetical index of V codes
    C. procedure codes
    D. table of drugs and chemicals

31. Omit code
    A. is a phrase that identifies procedures that might be included in the main procedure
    B. may require that the coder assign codes to individual components of a procedure
    C. identifies procedure codes for which Medicare will not provide reimbursement
    D. is an instructional notation used in the first volume of the ICD-9-CM code book

32. DSM-IV
    A. provides a system for classifying and coding of specimens
    B. allows for storage and data retrieval of pathology information
    C. is a statistical classification and glossary of mental disorders
    D. meets the needs of the ambulatory health care community

33. The discharged inpatient diagznostic statement "questionable coronary insufficiency" is
    A. coded as if confirmed
    B. not coded at all
    C. coded according to hospital policy
    D. coded at the coder's discretion

34. Assume there is a 40% difference between the payment made to a provider for the excision of a lesion that is .5 cm in length and one that is 3.2 cm in length; it would be important that the coder accurately
    A. document the size of the lesion in the patient's record
    B. screen precoded data submitted to the fiscal intermediary

    C. assign the CPT code number according to size of the lesion
    D. calculate the payment rate according to the size of the lesion

35. The general arrangement of the Surgery section in CPT-4 is according to
    A. specific name of the service or procedure performed on the patient
    B. anatomical site followed by the procedure or service performed
    C. name of the surgery, in alphabetic order by the name of the procedure
    D. name of the procedure or service, then categorized according to site

36. Which provide an explanation regarding the need for a special report?
    A. notes
    B. headings
    C. guidelines
    D. symbols

37. The coder who assigns an unlisted Surgery Section procedure code should
    A. request the physician to assign a code number for future use on the claim form
    B. include a copy of the surgical report with the insurance claim form submitted
    C. highlight the CPT-4 surgery code number assigned on the insurance claim form
    D. suggest to the CPT-4 that a new code be developed for future use

38. The coder would assign a code for the application of a cast when it is
    A. part of the initial fracture treatment
    B. considered a replacement procedure
    C. performed by an orthopedic specialist
    D. assisted by a medical assistant

39. Surgical destruction of a lesion would include all of the following EXCEPT:
    A. electrocautery
    B. cryosurgery
    C. laser
    D. debridement

40. The outpatient classification system developed by CMS to replace the ASC list is known as
    A. APCs
    B. DRGs
    C. RUGs
    D. RVUs

41. The case-mix system used for long-term care is known as
    A. activities of daily living (ADLs)
    B. resource utilization groups (RUGs)
    C. diagnostic related groups (DRGs)
    D. Medicare fee schedule

42. The _____ is the computer software program that is utilized to assign the appropriate DRGs according to the patient's principal and secondary diagnoses and principal procedure.
    A. grouper
    B. Coding Clinic
    C. case-mix
    D. encoder

43. Which severity of illness system abstracts clinical findings from the health record within 24 hours of hospitalization of ICU patients?
    A. AIM
    B. APACHE II
    C. ATLAS/MedisGroups
    D. Medicare Mortality Predictor System

44. _____ is a severity of illness system that uses data from the UB–92 along with a Q-Scale that assigns a score.
    A. Acuity Index Method (AIM)
    B. Computerized Severity Index (CSI)
    C. Disease Staging
    D. Acute Physiology and Chronic Health Evaluation II (APACHE II)

45. _____ indicates that the code is unspecified.
    A. NEC
    B. LOS
    C. NOS
    D. None of the above

46. Melinda is a coder and when she selects a principal diagnosis code that is NOS or unspecified, what should her next step be in the coding process?
    A. submit a special report and attach it to the insurance claim form
    B. ask the physician for a more specific diagnosis before assigning the code
    C. assign the unspecified code anyways
    D. select another code that is similar to avoid using the unspecified code

47. Where in the ICD-9-CM coding manual would you locate the Neoplasm Table?
    A. Volume I
    B. Volume II
    C. Volume III
    D. None of the above

48. You are coding and notice that the health record documents an error in dosage. What should you code this as?
    A. accidental ingestion
    B. poisoning
    C. overdose
    D. adverse effect

49. Manganese toxicity 985.2 + E866.4 would be classified in ICD-9-CM as a(n)
    A. accidental ingestion
    B. poisoning
    C. overdose
    D. adverse effect

50. When coding fractures, when there is no indication if the fracture is open or closed, code the condition as
    A. closed
    B. open
    C. unspecified
    D. other

51. A patient is treated at Milford Hospital and the diagnostic statement reads "Dislocation and fracture of right olecranon process." How would you code this condition?
    A. code the fracture of the olecranon process only
    B. code both the dislocation and fracture
    C. code the dislocation of the olecranon process only
    D. code fracture of the arm unspecified

52. When a foreign body is associated with an open wound, it is coded as:
    A. foreign body, then by site
    B. contusion
    C. open wound, complicated by site
    D. injury, superficial

53. A patient has first- and second-degree burns of the forearm. The coding sequence would be as follows:
    A. first-degree burn, forearm; second-degree burn, forearm
    B. second-degree burn, forearm
    C. second-degree burn, forearm; first-degree burn, forearm
    D. third-degree burn, forearm

DIRECTIONS: Questions 54–56 refer to the following case study. The patient was admitted on July 21 for chest pain. He was subsequently diagnosed with a urinary tract infection caused by Proteus and placed on Bactrim DS. The patient has a past history of small cell lung ca, status postchemotherapy and x-ray therapy; he also has a history of cardiomyopathy, prostate cancer, left bundle branch block, aortic aneurysm (for which the patient underwent surgical repair on May 1), esophagitis, and tobacco abuse. Physical examination revealed blood pressure of 116/82 and was positive for decreased breath sounds diffusely in the lungs; heart had distant heart sounds with S1 and S2; no S3. On admission, electrocardiogram revealed sinus bradycardia with frequent premature atrial contractions. Chest x-ray showed left upper lobe mass. Episodic chest pain continued throughout the admission, but was not associated with feeding or ambulation. Cardiac catheterization was performed on July 23. The patient wished to go home immediately following this procedure and the attending physician was agreeable. No clear etiology for chest pain was determined; the possibilities included: small pulmonary emboli, pain from metastatic disease, or gastroesophageal reflux.

54. Identify the principal diagnosis.
    A. Chest pain, unclear etiology
    B. Small cell lung carcinoma
    C. Left bundle branch block
    D. Urinary tract infection

55. Identify the principal procedure.
    A. Cardiac catheterization
    B. Chemotherapy
    C. Electrocardiogram
    D. Urinalysis with C&S

56. Identify the comorbidity.
    A. Aortic aneurysm
    B. Chest pain, unclear etiology
    C. Hypertension
    D. Urinary tract infection

57. Which of the following would not be a valid principal diagnosis code?
    A. V22.0 Supervision of normal first pregnancy
    B. V58.0 Radiotherapy
    C. V58.3 Attention to surgical dressings and sutures
    D. V10.3 History of malignant neoplasm, breast

58. When coding poisonings, what is the correct sequencing of codes?
    A. poisoning, manifestation, Table of Drugs and Chemicals E code
    B. manifestation, poisoning, Table of Drugs and Chemicals E code
    C. poisoning, E code
    D. manifestation, Table of Drugs and Chemicals E code

59. A star or asterisk (*) is utilized in the CPT manual to indicate
    A. a new code number
    B. a revised code number
    C. a revision in the text with the guidelines and instructions
    D. the code is not a part of a surgical package

60. A patient is seen in the Emergency Room complaining of lower abdominal pain and blood in the urine. A urinalysis done revealed numerous white and red blood cells and bacteria. A broad-spectrum antibiotic was prescribed with the diagnosis of "R/O UTI." The principal diagnosis is
    A. lower abdominal pain
    B. UTI
    C. hematuria
    D. R/O UTI

61. A patient is admitted to the hospital for follow-up examination (V67.0) for surgery performed previously. The patient has a history of breast cancer (V10.3). Diagnostic studies reveal metastasis to the brain (198.3). The proper coding sequence would be:
    V67.0 (Follow-up examination following surgery)
    V10.3 (History of breast cancer)
    174.9 (breast cancer, primary)
    198.3 (neoplasm, brain, secondary)
    A. V67.0, 174.9, 198.3, V10.3
    B. 198.3, 174.9, V67.0, V10.3
    C. 198.3, V67.0, V10.3
    D. 174.9, V67.0, V10.3

62. A patient is admitted to the hospital for anemia and is complaining of lethargy and nausea due to chemotherapy. The patient has prostate cancer. The patient is given a blood transfusion for the anemia and was discharged home from the hospital. The principal diagnosis in this case would be the
    A. anemia
    B. prostate cancer
    C. lethargy
    D. nausea

63. The instrument utilized to collect standardized SNF patient data is known as the
    A. case-mix analysis
    B. severity of illness
    C. clinical pertinence review
    D. resident assessment instrument (RAI)

64. The minimum core of patient information that is collected on the face sheet of skilled nursing facility patients is known as the
    A. problem list
    B. SOAP note
    C. Minimum Data Set 2.0 (MDS)
    D. Resource Utilization Groups III (RUGs III)

65. The first step in determining the correct Evaluation & Management code is based on what three factors?
    A. history, physical, medical decision making
    B. place of service, type of service, and patient status
    C. new patient, established patient, outpatient or inpatient
    D. counseling, coordination of care, nature of presenting problem

DIRECTIONS: Questions 66–69 refer to the following case study. The patient was admitted on June 22 with abdominal pain. She has a history of allergy to Sulfa. Past history reveals periumbilical hernia repair 10 years ago and right groin hernia repair 15 years ago. Present illness revealed that the patient developed abdominal pain 2 days prior to admission, located in the mid-upper abdomen. She denied association with positional changes. She did note increased urinary frequency and was advised to take Ciprofloxacin the day prior to admission for possible urinary tract infection. The patient arrived in the emergency department for further evaluation. The patient reports increased psychosocial stresses at home and notes consuming large amounts of beer, about five beers per night during the week prior to admission. Physical examination revealed a tired-appearing female lying in bed in obvious discomfort. Abdomen was soft, positive bowel sounds, nontympanitic with mild upper abdominal tenderness, no rebound, no rigidity, no hepatosplenomegaly, no lymph nodes in the inguinal region, no bruits, no suprapubic tenderness. Lab data revealed negative urinalysis and negative urine culture. Abdominal scan with contrast showed focal fatty infiltrative liver. The abdominal scan was basically unremarkable and the patient was observed overnight. Serial belly exams were unremarkable. The patient was discharged from the hospital to be followed in 1 week. Condition at discharge was stable; the patient was encouraged to taper her alcohol use and follow-up regarding that issue was recommended.

66. Identify the principal diagnosis.
    A. Abdominal pain
    B. Alcoholism
    C. Gastritis
    D. Fatty liver

67. Identify the principal procedure.
    A. Abdominal CT with contrast
    B. Hernia repair, periumbilical
    C. Serial belly examinations
    D. Urinalysis with urine culture

68. Identify the comorbidity.
    A. Abdominal pain
    B. Periumbilical hernia
    C. Psychosocial stress
    D. None of these

69. Identify the complication.
    A. Abdominal pain
    B. Psychosocial stress
    C. Urinary tract infection
    D. None of these

70. The key components of E/M service is based on what three factors?
    A. history, physical, medical decision making
    B. type of service, place of service, and patient status
    C. history, physical examination, contributing factors
    D. counseling, coordination of care, nature of presenting problem

71. The various elements that include chief complaint (CC), history of present illness (HPI), review of systems (ROS) and past/family and/or social history (PFSH) would be considered what key component when determining E&M code assignment?

A. history

B. physical examination

C. medical decision making

D. contributing factors

72. You are a coder assigning the correct E/M code for a patient record. You are looking at the patient record for the following information: the number of diagnoses or management options, amount or complexity of data to review, and the risk of complication or death if the condition goes untreated. What key component in E/M code assignment does this fall under?

    A. history

    B. physical examination

    C. contributing factors

    D. medical decision making

DIRECTIONS: Questions 73–76 refer to the following case study. The patient is admitted August 3 with a past history of hypertension, coronary artery disease, hypercholesterolemia, and acute esophagogastritis. He had an inferior wall myocardial infarction last March with 100% occlusion of the right coronary artery and underwent coronary angioplasty of the right coronary artery with reduction of lesion to 10%. During cardiac rehabilitation, he was noted to have prolonged ventricular tachycardia, which was essentially asymptomatic. Repeat cardiac catheterization on an outpatient basis in June revealed right coronary artery occlusion of 50%. During this current admission, electrocardiogram revealed right bundle branch block. Physical examination revealed blood pressure of 156/92, heart rate of 61, respiratory rate of 20, and oxygen saturation of 96% on room air. Patient is admitted for observation, initiation of Amiodarone therapy for ventricular tachycardia, and plans for implantable cardioverter defibrillator placement. During this admission, the patient did well and had no episodes of ventricular tachycardia. On August 6, the patient underwent placement of implantable cardioverter defibrillator without incident. A small hematoma at the insertion site was noted the day after the procedure, but it was otherwise clear. The patient was discharged August 8.

73. Identify the principal diagnosis.

    A. Coronary artery disease

    B. Myocardial infarction, old

    C. Right bundle branch block

    D. Ventricular tachycardia

74. Identify the principal procedure.

    A. Repeat cardiac catheterization procedure

    B. Coronary angioplasty of the right coronary artery

    C. Implantable cardioverter defibrillator placement

    D. Incision and drainage of insertion site hematoma

75. Identify the comorbidity.

    A. Coronary artery disease

    B. Malignant hypertension

    C. Myocardial infarction, old

    D. Ventricular tachycardia

76. Identify the complication.

    A. Coronary artery disease

    B. Hematoma, insertion site

    C. Malignant hypertension

    D. Ventricular tachycardia

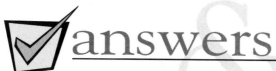

answers & rationales

1.

B. A medical nomenclature is a systematic listing of names. An example of a hospital-specific nomenclature would be SNDO. A classification groups similar information together. An example of this would be ICD-9-CM (Abdelhak, pp. 230–231; Johns, p. 292).

2.

B. Answer A is the definition of *NEC;* answer C defines *See Category;* and answer D defines *Notes* (Brown, pp. 11–18).

3.

C. NOS or *not otherwise specified* is virtually the equivalent of *unspecified.* Answer A is fabricated; answer B defines *NEC;* and answer D explains *includes* notes (Brown, pp. 11–19).

4.

A. Myocardial infarction, for example, would be located under *infarction* (the condition) rather than under *myocardium* (the site or topography). Morphology refers to structure and is used only in coding neoplasms. The chapters in Volume 1 are generally arranged according to body system. Subterms in Volume 2 provide the site (Brown, p. 6).

5.

A. In the first example, both acute conditions would be coded as if they were confirmed diagnoses. In the second example, both the depressive reaction and the hypothyroidism would be coded (Brown, pp. 19–21).

6.

B. The AMA revises and publishes annual versions of the CPT-4 manual (Smith, p. 1).

7.

B. The modifier can be submitted in the two-digit or five-digit format, as required by the insurance company (i.e., 19160-50 or 19160, 09950) (Smith, p. 18).

8.

D. The portion of the code prior to the semicolon is the common part of all codes in the series; thus the interpretation is answer D (Smith, pp. 14–15).

9.

C. The incision and drainage of the simple hematoma represents the major service performed for the patient during the visit. If the patient had also received a comprehensive history and physical examination, the code assignment would be 10140 and 99204 (CPT-4, p. 49).

10.

C. Complications that require additional services are coded according to the service provided. (Abdelhak, p. 240; Johns, pp. 370–371).

11.

B. The student should know the contents of each of the three volumes of ICD-9-CM (Abdelhak, p. 59; Johns, p. 294).

12.

D. "Use additional code" used to have the phrase "if desired" attached to it. Many code books have revised this instruction to delete "if desired." This is a mandatory instruction that coders must follow in the assignment of ICD-9-CM diagnosis codes (Brown, pp. 11–19).

13.

B. NEC or "not elsewhere classifiable" (or "not elsewhere classified") differs from NOS in that NEC refers to insufficient information in the Alphabetic Index or to the lack of a more specific subdivision in the Tabular Lists to classify a statement containing sufficient or greater detail. In other words, the problem is with the ICD-9-CM codes, not practitioner documentation. NOS refers to a lack of sufficient detail in the diagnostic or procedural statement; the problem is with insufficient documentation in the record for coding purposes (Brown, pp. 11–19).

14.

A. Eponyms refer to terms named after a person or place (e.g., Holmes). AIDS is an acronym for acquired immune deficiency syndrome. An acronym is a word comprised of initials. Miscarriage is a lay term for abortion. A carcinoma is a malignant growth (Brown, p. 49).

15.

A. Ruled-out conditions would not be assigned a code. If the condition is stated as "rule out," code it as if it were established. Remember that the rule changes for outpatient diagnoses stated as "rule out"; code the symptom(s) documented in the record (Brown, pp. 40–41).

16.

A. The coder should refer to pathology results on the patient prior to assigning an excision of lesion code (Smith, p. 70).

17.

A. Guidelines are located at the beginning of each of the six sections of CPT-4. The Introduction is lo-cated just before the Evaluation and Management section and instructions in the use of CPT-4 are contained within the Introduction (Smith, pp. 21, 22, 24).

18.

D. If the coder cannot determine the correct code assignment by referring to the name of the procedure in the CPT-4 index, the anatomic site can be referenced. In addition, the coder can refer to an eponym, a synonym, or an abbreviation in the CPT-4 index to determine the code assignment (Smith, p. 22).

19.

C. A code that indicates "interpretation and report only" means that a different provider performed the electrocardiogram (Buck, p. 341).

20.

B. Annual revisions of CPT-4 contain altered procedure descriptions for certain codes, indicated by the triangle symbol next to the code number (Smith, p. 2).

21.

A. CMS is the administrative agency located in the Department of HHS that provides uniform reporting and statistical data collection of medical procedures, supplies, products, and services (Smith, p. 2).

22.

C. Answer A describes the use of the colon; answer B describes the use of braces; and answer D is fabricated (Brown, p. 15).

23.

B. When the term *and* appears in an ICD-9-CM code title, it is interpreted as *and* or *or*. According to the American Hospital Association, "for example, code 415.1x in Volume 1 includes pulmonary embolism and/or pulmonary infarction" (Brown, p. 17).

24.

D. Acute and chronic episodes of a disease are often quite different in terms of their etiology, treatment, and prognosis. They should be coded according to the subentries in the alphabetic index (Brown, pp. 41–42).

25.

B. CPT-4 is updated annually with codes added and deleted, and code descriptions changed. To obtain proper reimbursement, it is necessary that an up-to-date version of CPT-4 be utilized. If a deleted code is submitted to an insurance company or fiscal intermediary, it will either be changed or the claim returned to the provider for correction (slowing down payment to the provider) (CPT-4, p. xv).

26.

A. When the provider attempts to restore a fracture or dislocation, regardless of type, it is referred to as manipulation or reduction (Smith, p. 80).

27.

D. All surgery codes include the "operation per se, local infiltration, metacarpal/digital block or topical anesthesia when used, and normal, uncomplicated follow-up care" (Buck, p. 132; Smith, pp. 58–59).

28.

C. Code 59426 refers to the patient who receives care prior to delivery. Code 59400–22 includes unusual services, a modifier that is not applicable in this case. Code 59430 refers to the patient who receives care after delivery (Smith, p. 58).

29.

C. When assigning a surgery code, be sure to review the record for the surgical approach, as this will indicate proper code assignment (Brown, p. 50).

30.

A. The table of drugs and chemicals and an indexed reference to V codes within the main body of the al-phabetical index are in Volume 2. Procedure codes are in Volume 3 (Brown, pp. 4–6).

31.

A. "Omit code" is used in Volume 3 of ICD-9-CM to identify services or procedures that are a component of a larger service or procedure; thus, the instruction to omit code is provided (Brown, p. 50).

32.

C. Answer A refers to SNOP (Systematized Nomenclature of Pathology); answer B refers to SNOMED (Systematized Nomenclature of Medicine); and answer D refers to ICHPPC (International Classification of Health Problems in Primary Care). DSM-IV (Diagnostic and Statistical Manual of Mental Disorders) is an expansion of the mental disorders section of ICD (Abdelhak, p. 256; Johns, p. 308).

33.

A. Suspected, questionable, likely, or possible diagnoses for discharged inpatient cases are coded as if confirmed (Brown, p. 73).

34.

C. CPT-4 categorizes codes for the excision of a benign lesion and the excision of a malignant lesion under separate headings. There is additional categorization according to the location and size of the lesion. Therefore, the coder must determine the correct code assignment based on these criteria (Smith, p. 70).

35.

B. The Surgery Section is subdivided by body system, then by anatomic site, then by category of procedure (with the exception of the Maternity Care and Delivery subsection) (Smith, p. 57).

36.

C. Guidelines are located at the beginning of each CPT-4 section and provide clarification as to modifiers to be used with section codes, need for a special report with submission of an unlisted procedure code, etc. (CPT-4, p. xiv).

37.

B. Unlisted procedure or service codes are assigned when a specific code is not found in CPT-4; along with this code, a special report is submitted to the insurance company (Buck, pp. 16–18).

38.

B. Cast applications or strappings are coded when performed as "a replacement procedure during or after the period of follow-up care, or when the cast application or strapping is an initial service performed without a restorative treatment or procedure(s) to stabilize or protect a fracture, injury, or dislocation and/or to afford comfort to a patient" (CPT-4, p. 99).

39.

D. Different methods of destruction are not coded separately but are categorized under the heading, Destruction. Debridement is actually entitled Excision - Debridement and is found in a subheading under Skin, Subcutaneous and Accessory Structures (CPT-4, pp. 51, 56).

40.

A. APCs stands for ambulatory payment groups, which was to be a PPS to cover outpatient services that utilizes ICD-9-CM and CPT procedure codes (Buck, p. 561; Johns, p. 367).

41.

B. Resource utilization groups are a case-mix management system that uses information from a minimum data set for long-term care patients. ADLs is information abstracted along with clinical characteristics of the patient, which is entered into the minimum data set for long-term settings (Abdelhak, p. 258; Buck, p. 560).

42.

A. The DRG grouper is a software program that follows a logic sequence that determines the DRG for each patient according to the principal diagnosis, comorbities, complications, and principal procedure. An encoder is a computerized ICD-9-CM and/or CPT program that assists in assigning diagnosis and procedure codes (Abdelhak, pp. 238–240; Rogers, p. 74).

43.

B. APACHE stands for Acute Physiology and Chronic Health Evaluation and is a severity of illness system utilized for ICU patients (Abdelhak, pp. 257–258).

44.

C. Disease Staging is a type of severity of illness system that is utilized in hospitals from data from the UB-92 (Abdelhak, pp. 257–258).

45.

C. NOS stands for not otherwise specified and is used when the physician's documentation is not specific (Brown, pp. 14, 36).

46.

B. According to the Official Guidelines for Coding and Reporting, "Use 'unspecified' (NOS) when the information at hand does not permit either a more specific or 'other' code assignment." The coder should consult the attending physician to get a more specific principal diagnosis for proper DRG assignment (Brown, p. 378).

47.

B. The Neoplasm Table is located in Volume II Index to Diseases in the ICD-9-CM coding book (Brown, p. 288).

48.

B. A documentation error in recording of medication dosage is classified as a poisoning in the ICD-9-CM coding manual (Brown, p. 335).

49.

D. According to Brown, "A diagnostic statement of toxic effect, toxicity, or intoxication due to a prescription drug such as digitalis or lithium without any further qualification usually refers to an adverse effect of a correctly administered prescription drug" (Brown, p. 335).

50.

A. When there is no indication as to whether the fracture is stated as open or closed, code the condition as closed (Brown, p. 313).

51.

A. If there is a patient who suffers from a dislocation and fracture, the dislocation code is included in the fracture code (Brown, p. 320).

52.

C. According to the Official Coding Guidelines, when a foreign body is associated with a fracture, it is coded as open wound, complicated by site (Brown, p. 313).

53.

C. When sequencing codes for burns, you code to the highest degree burn first and if there are multiple degrees of burn of the same site, you code to the highest degree only. Therefore, second-degree burn of the forearm would be the only code in this scenario (Brown, p. 330).

54.

A. The attending physician in this case was unable to clearly identify the cause of the chest pain, so it is identified as principal diagnosis. Principal diagnosis is defined as "the condition established after study to be chiefly responsible for occasioning the admission of the patient to the hospital for care" (Abdelhak, p. 235; Johns, p. 370).

55.

A. The chemotherapy was performed during a previous admission. The electrocardiogram and urinalysis with culture and sensitivity are lab tests. Thus, the cardiac catheterization most closely meets the definition of principal procedure. Principal procedure is defined as "one that was performed for definitive treatment rather than one performed for diagnostic or exploratory purposes, or was necessary to take care of a complication; if there appear to be two procedures that are principal, then the one most related to the principal diagnosis would be selected as the principal procedure" (Brown, pp. 47–48).

56.

D. The aortic aneurysm was dealt with during a previous admission as mentioned in the past history of the case study. There does not appear to be documentation of hypertension during this admission. "Chest pain, unclear etiology" is the principal diagnosis. Comorbidity is defined as "a condition existing at the time of hospitalization which has potential for affecting the course of illness or medical care provided." The Uniform Hospital Discharge Data Set refers to secondary diagnoses as "other diagnoses" and defines them as "all conditions that co-exist at the time of admission, that develop subsequently, or that affect the treatment received and/or length of stay; diagnoses that relate to an earlier episode which have no bearing on the current hospital stay are to be excluded" (Brown, pp. 22–25).

57.

D. History codes can only be used as additional diagnoses (Brown, pp. 66–67).

58.

A. When coding poisonings, you code poisoning code first, then the effect and the E code from the Table and Drugs and Chemicals table (Brown, p. 335).

59.

D. Starred procedures are minor surgeries that do not include the surgery package concept, which includes the preoperative and postoperative care that is routine to the care provided (Smith, p. 61).

60.

A. According to the Diagnostic Coding and Reporting Guidelines for Outpatient Services (Hospital-Based and Physician-Office), Revised October 1, 1995, "Do not code diagnoses documented as 'probable,' 'suspected,' 'questionable,' 'rule out,' or 'working diagnosis.' Rather code to the highest degree of certainty . . ." (Brown, p. 396; Buck, p. 601).

61.

C. According to the official coding guidelines, "Any mention of extension, invasion, or metastasis to a nearby structure or organ or to a distant site is coded as a secondary malignant neoplasm is designated as the principal diagnosis even though the primary malignancy is still present" (Brown, p. 382).

62.

A. According to official coding guidelines, "When the admission is for management of an anemia associated with chemotherapy or radiotherapy and the only treatment is for the anemia, the anemia is designated as the principal diagnosis followed by the appropriate code(s) for the malignancy" (Brown, p. 382).

63.

D. The assessment instrument is called the RAI and includes the Minimum Data Set 2.0 (MDS) (Johns, 373).

64.

C. The Minimum Data Set is the instrument used to collect information, including patient demographic and activities of daily living, etc., for skilled nursing facilities (Johns, p. 374).

65.

B. The first thing you must consider when selecting the proper E/M code is place of service (office, hospital, ER, nursing home). The second factor in code assignment is type of service (consultation, admission, newborn care, and office visit). The third factor in E/M code assignment is patient status (new patient, established patient, outpatient and inpatient) (Buck, pp. 30–31).

66.

A. There was no diagnosis of alcoholism, gastritis, or fatty liver (cirrhosis) specifically documented in this case. It would be appropriate to question the physician to determine whether something other than abdominal pain could be selected as principal diagnosis; however, it would be necessary for the physician to document the selected diagnosis (and it would also need to have been documented throughout the record). Principal diagnosis is defined as "the condition established after study to be chiefly responsible for occasioning the admission of the patient to the hospital for care" (Abdelhak, p. 235; Johns, p. 370).

67.

A. The hernia repair was performed during a previous admission. Serial belly examinations involve physical examination of the patient's abdomen and would not be considered a procedure. The urinalysis with urine culture is a lab exam. The best response would be the Abdominal CT with contrast. It would be important to determine whether the facility for which you work collects such data, however. Principal procedure is defined as "one that was performed for definitive treatment rather than one performed for diagnostic or exploratory purposes, or was necessary to take care of a complication; if there appear to be two procedures that are principal, then the one most related to the principal diagnosis would be selected as the principal procedure" (Abdelhak, p. 87; Johns, pp. 370–371).

68.

D. Abdominal pain is the principal diagnosis. The periumbilical hernia was treated during a previous admission. While psychosocial stress could possibly be considered a comorbidity, there is no documentation that this problem was treated (i.e., either with medication or therapy). Thus, there is no evidence of any comorbidities for this case. Comorbidity is defined as "a condition existing at the time of hospitalization which has potential for affecting the course of illness or medical care provided." The UHDDS refers to secondary diagnoses as "other diagnoses" and defines them as "all conditions that co-exist at the time of admission, that develop subsequently, or that affect the treatment received and/or length of stay; diagnoses that relate to an earlier episode which have no bearing on the current hospital stay are to be excluded" (Abdelhak, p. 240; Johns, pp. 370–371).

69.

D. The abdominal pain is the principal diagnosis in this case; psychosocial stress was not treated during the admission; and the urinary tract infection was ruled out via lab tests. Thus, none of these must be selected as the answer. Complication is defined as "a condition arising during the hospitalization that modifies the course of the patient's illness or the medical care required" (Abdelhak, p. 240; Johns, pp. 370–371).

70.

A. The key components of history, physical examination, and medical decision making "reflect the clinical information that is recorded by the physician in the patient's medical record" (Buck, p. 32).

71.

A. There are four elements of a history, which include chief complaint, history of present illness, review of systems, and past, family, and/or social history (Buck, p. 33).

72.

D. The key component of medical decision making is based on the complexity of the patient's condition for which the physician has to factor in these elements: diagnoses and management options, data to review, and the level of risk of presenting problem(s) (Buck, p. 43).

73.

D. The inferior wall MI (myocardial infarction) occurred previous to this admission. The right bundle branch block (RBBB) is an ECG (electrocardiogram) finding. The coronary artery disease was the principal diagnosis for the admission during which angioplasty of the right coronary artery was performed. Thus, the ventricular tachycardia is the principal diagnosis (note that ICD placement was performed during this current admission to resolve this problem). Principal diagnosis is defined as "the condition established after study to be chiefly responsible for occasioning the admission of the patient to the hospital for care" (Abdelhak, p. 235; Brown, p. 19).

74.

C. The cardiac catheterization was performed on an outpatient basis in June; coronary angioplasty was performed during a previous admission to resolve the coronary artery disease; and there is no mention of an incision and drainage of the hematoma being performed during this admission. The ICD (implantable cardioverter-defibrillator) placement was performed during this admission to resolve the ventricular tachycardia problem. Principal procedure is defined as "one that was performed for definitive treatment rather than one performed for diagnostic or exploratory purposes, or was necessary to take care of a complication; if there appear to be two procedures that are principal, then the one most related to the principal diagnosis would be selected as the principal procedure" (Abdelhak, p. 87; Brown, p. 47).

75.

C. There is no documentation of malignant hypertension, although the patient's blood pressure is elevated upon physical examination. The ventricular tachycardia is the principal diagnosis. The coronary artery disease, although obviously a coexisting condition, did not receive treatment in this case. Thus, the old myocardial infarction would be the comorbidity. Comorbidity is defined as "a condition existing at the time of hospitalization which has potential for affecting the course of illness or medical care provided." The UHDDS refers to secondary diagnoses as "other diagnoses" and defines them as "all conditions that co-exist at the time of admission, that develop subsequently, or that affect the treatment received and/or length of stay; diagnoses that relate to an earlier episode which have no bearing on the current hospital stay are to be excluded" (Abdelhak, p. 240; Brown, p. 22).

76.

B. The hematoma, insertion site is the only condition that arose during the patient's stay. Complication is defined as "a condition arising during the hospitalization that modifies the course of the patient's illness or the medical care required" (Abdelhak, p. 240; Brown, p. 22).

4 Reimbursement Methodologies

objectives

After completion of this chapter, the student will be able to:

➤ Explain the prospective payment systems.

➤ Describe the components of the DRG system.

➤ Explain the purpose of PROs.

➤ Explain the RBRVS system.

➤ Discuss issues related to Medicare fraud and abuse.

➤ Identify the major components of managed care and capitation.

➤ Distinguish between the various managed care organizations.

➤ Describe the structure of the APC system.

➤ Develop an understanding of the billing and insurance claim cycle and procedures for the different health care settings and managed care.

DIRECTIONS (Questions 1–46): Each of the questions or incomplete statements below is followed by suggested answers or completions. Select the **best** answer in each case.

---

1. The payment system utilized for physician's services that was developed as a result of the Omnibus Budget Reconciliation Act of 1989 is known as
   A. RBRVS
   B. ASC
   C. APGs
   D. CPT-4

2. According to the RBRVS, the relative value unit (RVU) is based on all of the following EXCEPT:
   A. physician work
   B. overhead expense
   C. malpractice expense
   D. education

3. A major revision of the Omnibus Budget Reconciliation Act of 1990 (OBRA), Public Law 101-239 included the establishment of
   A. relative value units
   B. physician fee schedule
   C. DRG system
   D. APGs

4. Until 2001, the Centers for Medicare and Medicaid Services was known as what organization?
   A. Centers for Disease Control (CDC)
   B. Health Care Financing Administration (HCFA)
   C. Joint Commission on the Accreditation of Healthcare Organizations (JCAHO)
   D. American Medical Association (AMA)

5. The relative value units that are assigned for payment of physician services using CPT codes are based on
   A. age of patient
   B. case-mix
   C. geographic area
   D. sex of patient

6. Who is responsible for developing and monitoring the work plan that outlines guidelines for identification of Medicare fraud and abuse?
   A. CMS
   B. AMA
   C. HCFA
   D. OIG

7. What was developed by CMS to replace the ASC list and designed to be a prospective payment system for ambulatory care?
   A. APCs
   B. DRGs
   C. RUGs
   D. RVUs

8. Which of the following measures the type and categories of patients treated by the healthcare facility?
   A. case-mix systems
   B. resource utilization groups (RUGs)
   C. diagnostic related groups (DRGs)
   D. all of the above

9. The case-mix system used for long-term care is known as
   A. activities of daily living (ADLs)
   B. resource utilization groups (RUGs)
   C. diagnostic related groups (DRGs)
   D. Medicare fee schedule

10. The _____ is the computer software program that is utilized to assign the appropriate DRGs according to the patient's princi-

pal and secondary diagnoses and principal procedure.
- A. grouper
- B. MDC
- C. case-mix
- D. severity of illness

11. Which insurance claim is utilized for physician office claims?
- A. UB-92
- B. HCFA-1450
- C. HCFA-1500
- D. UB-82

12. Which insurance claim is utilized for inpatient hospital claims?
- A. UB-92
- B. HCFA-1451
- C. HCFA-1500
- D. UB-82

13. Diagnosis-related groups are organized into how many MDCs?
- A. 23
- B. 24
- C. 25
- D. 26

14. The DRG system was implemented in what year?
- A. 1990
- B. 1983
- C. 1965
- D. 1973

15. Under the acute care prospective payment system (DRGs), how many DRGs does the list consist of?
- A. 510
- B. 515
- C. 519
- D. 523

16. The Balanced Budget Act of 1997 authorized implementation of a Medicare prospective payment system (PPS) for outpatient services in October 2001 known as
- A. Ambulatory Payment Classification (APCs)
- B. Outpatient Prospective Payment System (OPPS)
- C. Case-Mix Groups (CMGs)
- D. Ambulatory Payment Groups (APGs)

17. CMS developed and implemented the _____ in 1996 to establish correct coding practices to improve appropriate payment. This is known as the
- A. Compliance Program Guidance
- B. Correct Coding Initiative (CCI)
- C. Code of Federal Regulations (CFR)
- D. Minimum Data Set for Post Acute Care (MDS-PAC)

18. The home health prospective payment system (HHPPS) is based on what data for patient assessments?
- A. MDS 2.0
- B. HESIS
- C. UHDDS
- D. OASIS

19. The Office of Inspector General (OIG) of the Department of Health and Human Services (HHS) published the _____ to develop controls to prevent fraud and abuse of health care plans.
- A. Compliance Program Guidance
- B. Correct Coding Initiative (CCI)
- C. Code of Federal Regulations (CFR)
- D. Minimum Data Set for Post Acute Care (MDS-PAC)

20. The type of reimbursement methodology where payment of patient services is determined before the service is delivered refers to which type of payment system?
    A. retrospective payment system
    B. fee-for-service payment system
    C. prospective payment system
    D. managed fee-for-service system

21. Federal legislation that attempts to eliminate unbundling or other inappropriate reporting of CPT codes is known as the
    A. Compliance Program Guidance
    B. Correct Coding Initiative (CCI)
    C. Federal False Claims Amendment Act
    D. Health Insurance Portability and Accountability Act (HIPAA)

22. The organization who is under contract with the government that handles claims under Medicare Part A and/or B is known as the:
    A. peer review organization (PRO)
    B. Medigap (MG)
    C. Centers for Medicare and Medicaid Services (CMS)
    D. fiscal intermediary (FI)

23. Medicare Part B covers all of the following EXCEPT:
    A. outpatient medical and surgical services and supplies
    B. clinical laboratory tests
    C. home health care
    D. inpatient medical and surgical services and supplies

24. The government-sponsored program that provides health care insurance coverage to those age 65 or older, certain disabled people, those requiring kidney dialysis, and kidney transplant patients is
    A. TRICARE
    B. CHAMPVA
    C. Medicaid
    D. Medicare

25. The government-sponsored program that provides hospital and medical services for dependents of active service personnel and retired service personnel, as well as dependents of members who died on active duty, is known as
    A. TRICARE
    B. CHAMPVA
    C. Medicaid
    D. Medicare

26. The system of payment used by managed care plans in which physicians and hospitals are paid on a fixed, per capita amount for each patient and for hospitals on a per-member/per-month basis to cover costs of the plan is known as
    A. fee-for-service
    B. managed fee-for-service
    C. episode of care reimbursement
    D. capitation

27. The type of managed care organization where a group of facilities are contracted together to provide a comprehensive set of services that any patient may need and are recognized by the public as a combined operating entity is known as a
    A. Health Maintenance Organization (HMO)
    B. Preferred Provider Organization (PPO)
    C. Point of Service Plan (POS)
    D. Integrated Delivery System (IDS)

28. This document describes the services billed and includes a breakdown of how the payment was determined.
    A. HCFA-1500 claim form
    B. Explanation of Benefits (EOB)
    C. chargemaster
    D. encounter form

29. As supervisor of the file area, a new employee brings a health record to your attention because there is a document attached to the health record. This document contains patient information, areas to check off or diagnoses and procedures, and the patient's next appointment date. This form is known as the
   A. patient registration form
   B. Explanation of Benefits (EOB) form
   C. chargemaster form
   D. Authorization for Release of Information Form

30. Payment rates for each DRG are determined from an assigned relative weighting factor and the
   A. acute care facility's wage rate index calculation
   B. individual hospital's payment rate per case
   C. average resources required to treat patient cases
   D. regional/national adjusted standardized amount

31. What was the origin of the Medicare and Medicaid programs?
   A. Federal regulations passed by the Department of Health, Education, and Welfare
   B. Amendments to the Social Security Act of 1965, as passed by the U.S. Congress
   C. Federal regulations of the Social Security Administration, passed in 1965
   D. Federal legislation established via individual state ratification of the programs

32. The condition chiefly responsible for occasioning the admission of the patient to the hospital for care is called
   A. primary diagnosis
   B. principal diagnosis
   C. principle diagnosis
   D. provisional diagnosis

33. When selecting the major diagnostic category, you need to

   A. consider whether a procedure was performed
   B. identify the patient's date of birth and age
   C. review the patient's disposition upon discharge
   D. assign an ICD-9-CM code to the primary diagnosis

34. The DRG weight in a case is .5631; the payment rate is $3,027.00. Calculate the amount of money the hospital will receive as reimbursement for this case.
   A. $8,658.00
   B. $3,027.00
   C. $2,604.00
   D. $1,704.50

35. Who assigns the correct DRG under the Prospective Payment System?
   A. insurance carrier
   B. acute care facility
   C. health information coder
   D. fiscal intermediary

36. As a result of the war on poverty during the Johnson administration, socioeconomic needs were addressed via the implementation of the Medicare and Medicaid health care programs. What was the immediate impact?
   A. patient populations previously unable to pay for health care were now eligible for health care provided free of charge by physicians in the community
   B. individuals who previously were unable to pay for health care received care for which facilities and physicians were reimbursed by the government
   C. Congress authorized the investigation of the possible implementation of a prospective payment system to control spiraling health care costs
   D. the government required that private health insurance be provided to the population of the United States, regardless of a person's ability to pay for it

37. Why was the UHDDS implemented?
    A. to provide a reporting mechanism for the prospective payment system
    B. to create a uniform reporting mechanism for long-term care facilities
    C. to allow ambulatory and acute care facilities to compare health data
    D. to improve the uniformity and comparability of hospital discharge data

38. Select the sequence of steps needed to manually assign a diagnosis-related group.
    A. principal diagnosis, decision tree, major diagnostic category, diagnosis-related group
    B. principal diagnosis, major diagnostic category, decision tree, diagnosis-related group
    C. principal diagnosis, diagnosis-related group, major diagnostic category, decision tree
    D. principal diagnosis, major diagnostic category, diagnosis-related group, decision tree

39. Cases reimbursed according to DRGs that have a long length of stay or very high costs are termed
    A. long term
    B. outliers
    C. exceptions
    D. special

40. What is the function of the UB-92?
    A. compilation of health care statistics
    B. submission of hospital claims to Medicare
    C. provision of data to residency programs
    D. observance of the state's regulations

41. Why was the Prospective Payment System initially implemented?
    A. to place constraints on health care cost increases

    B. to force physicians to comply with federal regulations
    C. to assist hospitals in remaining viable (open for business)
    D. to accommodate the needs of long-term care facilities

42. Which could result if the physician doesn't select the principal diagnosis?
    A. patient is treated for the wrong condition during hospitalization
    B. facility receives incorrect reimbursement from the insurance company
    C. physician is sanctioned by the hospital for incorrect selection
    D. nothing would result as it is the primary diagnosis that is important

43. When the hospital receives a DRG payment that is greater than the cost of care provided, the facility
    A. retains the surplus funds
    B. reimburses Medicare
    C. is considered guilty of "DRG creep"
    D. absorbs the loss of payment

44. Which is the correct definition of principal procedure?
    A. a procedure done for therapeutic rather than diagnostic reasons
    B. the procedure most closely related to the surgeon's specialty
    C. a procedure done for diagnostic rather than therapeutic reasons
    D. a procedure most closely related to primary diagnosis

45. What is the goal of DRGs?
    A. to increase utilization of Medicare services in hospitals
    B. to increase hospital lengths of stay for Medicare patients

C. to reduce hospital lengths of stay and increase revenues

D. to reduce spending on the Medicare patient population

46. What is the dollar amount Medicare will pay for a physician service, which is calculated by multiplying it with the relative value unit?

A. case-mix

B. deductible

C. DRG

D. conversion factor

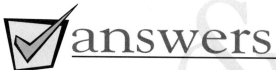

answers & rationales

1.

A. The Resource Based Relative Value System (RBRVS) is used for payment of physician's services (Abdelhak, p. 230; Buck, pp. 554–556; Smith, pp. 146–147).

2.

D. Physician work, practice expense (overhead), and malpractice expense are the standard relative values per procedure/service (Abdelhak, p. 230; Buck, p. 555; Smith, p. 148).

3.

B. The physician fee schedule is updated on April 15 of each year. The physician fee schedule is made up of RVUs for each service, a geographic adjustment factor, and a national conversion factor (Buck, pp. 554–555; Johns, pp. 373–374).

4.

B. HCFA is now known as Centers for Medicare and Medicaid Services (CMS) (Johns, p. 32).

5.

C. The relative value units are assigned payment according to considerations of geographic area for each of the three RVUs (work, overhead, malpractice) (Abdelhak, p. 624; Buck, p. 576).

6.

D. The Office of Inspector General (OIG) is responsible for the work plan that outlines the guidelines for identification of Medicare fraud and abuse. The CMS administers the Medicare program and establishes specific regulations in the *Medicare Carriers Manual (MCM)* for insurance carriers to follow. HCFA is now known as the CMS (Buck, p. 565).

7.

A. APCs stand for ambulatory payment classifications, which was to be a PPS to cover outpatient services that utilizes ICD-9-CM and CPT procedure codes (Johns, p. 367).

8.

D. According to Abdelhak, case-mix systems are a method used "which attempt to classify patients according to a common characteristic." RUGs and DRGs are both case-mix systems (pp. 257–258).

9.

B. Resource utilization groups are a case-mix management system that uses information from a minimum data set for long-term care patients. ADLs is information abstracted along with clinical characteristics of the patient, which is entered into the minimum data set for long-term settings (Abdelhak, p. 258).

10.

A. The DRG grouper is a software program that follows a logical sequence that determines the DRG for each patient according to the principal diagnosis, comorbidities, complications, and principal procedure (Abdelhak, pp. 238–240, Rogers, p. 74).

11.

C. The HCFA 1500 is the universal health insurance claim form that is used to obtain reimbursement for services provided by physicians and allied health professionals (Smith, pp. 4–6).

12.

A. ICD-9-CM codes are reported on the UB-92 form, which is used in hospitals (Buck, pp. 386–387).

13.

C. There are 25 major diagnostic categories that are used in the DRG decision tree process (Johns, p. 371).

14.

B. The DRG system, which is a prospective payment system, was implemented in hospitals in 1983 (Johns, p. 370).

15.

A. The CMS adjusts the Medicare DRG list every year and for fiscal year 2003, the list consists of 510 DRGs (Zeisset, p. 68).

16.

B. The Medicare/Medicaid Outpatient Prospective Payment System was implemented in October 2001, which is a PPS for outpatient services (Johns, p. 375).

17.

B. The CCI was implemented to correct coding errors to improve appropriate payment for Medicare Part B claims (Johns, pp. 396–397).

18.

D. OASIS stands for the Outcomes and Assessment Information Set and this data set is used to conduct patient assessments (Johns, p. 378).

19.

A. The compliance program guidance is published by the OIG of the Department of HHS to assist health care organizations to develop internal controls "that promote adherence to applicable federal and state law, and program requirements of federal, state and private health plans" (Johns, p. 398).

20.

C. In a prospective payment system, the amount for each service is predetermined for each service a patient may receive is already calculated before the service is rendered (Johns, p. 362).

21.

B. Medicare's CCI is implemented to eliminate inappropriate reporting of coding, that is unbundling of CPT codes (Fordney, p. 315).

22.

D. Fiscal intermediary is the organization that handles Medicare A and B claims, which is also known as a fiscal agent, a fiscal carrier, or a claims processor (Fordney, p. 320).

23.

D. According to the "Medicare & You 2003" website, Medicare Part B helps cover outpatient service and supplies, including outpatient diagnostic, clinical laboratory, ambulatory surgery center facility fees, and home health care (http://www.medicare.gov/publications/pubs/pdf/10050.pdf, p. 7).

24.

D. CHAMPVA covers spouses and children of veterans with total, permanent, service-connected disabilities, or of the surviving spouses and children of veterans who died. Medicaid provides benefits to indigent persons on welfare, aged individuals. TRICARE provides hospital and medical services for dependents of active service personnel and retired service personnel, as well as dependents of members who died on active duty (Abdelhak, pp. 23, 41; Fordney, p. 44; Johns, pp. 352–355).

25.

A. CHAMPVA covers spouses and children of veterans with total, permanent, service-connected disabilities, or of the surviving spouses and children of veterans who died. Medicaid provides benefits to indigent persons on welfare, aged individuals. TRICARE provides hospital and medical services for dependents of active service personnel and retired service personnel, as well as dependents of members who died on active duty (Fordney, p. 44, Abdelhak, pp. 23, 41; Johns, pp. 352–355).

26.

D. Capitation is used by managed care plans in which physicians and hospitals are paid on a fixed, per capita amount for each patient and for hospitals on a per-member/per-month basis to cover costs of the plan. In fee-for-service, a fee is charged for each service or procedure performed. Managed fee-for service uses a fee schedule, which is a listing of acceptable charges. Episode of care reimbursement uses the global surgical fee as the basis for payment (Fordney, p. 236).

27.

D. An HMO provides health services for a covered population after prepayment of a fixed premium. PPOs contract with providers that utilize a preferred network of providers. POS plans combine HMO and PPO concepts where the insured makes out-of-pocket cost options. The IDS is a group of facilities that contract together, which are owned, leased, and grouped together by long-term contracts (Fordney, 244; Johns, p. 355; Peden, p. 77).

28.

B. The EOB is the document that describes the services billed and includes a breakdown of how the payment was determined. The HCFA-1500 claim form is the insurance claim form, which is submitted to the insurance company for services/procedures performed. The chargemaster or encounter form, service slip, routine form, or superbill contains areas to check off or write diagnoses and procedures and is attached to the patient's chart at the patient's visit (Fordney, p. 60; Johns, pp. 391–392).

29.

C. The chargemaster form (or encounter form, service slip, routine form, superbill, or charge slip) contains areas to check off or write diagnoses and procedures and is attached to the patient's chart at the patient's visit. The EOB is the document that describes the services billed and includes a breakdown of how the payment was determined. The HCFA-1500 claim form is the insurance claim form, which is submitted to the insurance company for services/procedures performed. The patient registration form is filled out upon admission by the patient. The Authorization for Release of Information Form is signed by the patient before receiving any treatment, which gives authorization to release information to the insurance company (Fordney, p. 60; Johns, pp. 391–392).

30.

B. The payment rate for each DRG is based on the relative weighting factor, which represents the average resources required to care for cases in a particular DRG, and the individual hospital's payment rate per case, which is based on regional or national adjusted standardized amounts (considering the type of hospital). The wage rate index calculation is included in the calculation of the individual hospital's payment rate per case (Rogers, pp. 39–40).

31.

B. The amendments were added to the Social Security Act in 1965 as part of PL 89–97. Medicare (Title XVIII) and Medicaid (Title XIX) came into being as a result of these amendments (Abdelhak, pp. 8–9, 13).

32.

B. The principal diagnosis is the correct answer. The primary diagnosis is that which consumes the most resources. This is the diagnosis that was often captured first prior to implementation of the Prospective Payment System. Principle diagnosis is an incorrect spelling of the answer. Provisional diagnosis is the physician's working diagnosis (Abdelhak, pp. 85, 235; Johns, p. 370).

33.

A. Patients in each Major Diagnostic Category are subdivided into two groups depending on the presence or absence of qualifying surgery. It is important to have an understanding of the manual assignment of DRGs. Another resource is the chapter on Reimbursement located in Buck. There are several case examples of DRG assignments in this book (Abdelhak, pp. 238–239).

34.

D. Reimbursement is determined by multiplying the relative weighting factor of the DRG by the hospital's individual payment rate. There may be applicable deductible amounts that the patient must pay; these would be subtracted from the amount paid by Medicare (Abdelhak, p. 258; Johns, p. 371).

35.

D. The fiscal intermediary (FI), which may be a Blue Cross plan, a private insurance company, or other agency, assigns the inpatient DRG based on codes supplied by the hospital. While the FI processes and pays Medicare Part A (inpatient) claims, the contractor that processes claims under Medicare Part B is called a carrier (Abdelhak, pp. 40, 42).

36.

B. Health care access in the United States, prior to the implementation of Medicare and Medicaid, was provided through charity, philanthropy, and retrospective fee-for-service payment. If people became ill and could not pay for care, they either were treated on a charitable basis or did not have access to health care (Abdelhak, pp. 8–9; Johns, p. 255).

37.

D. The UHDDS defines diagnoses and procedures to be captured for reimbursement purposes (i.e., principal diagnosis, comorbidity, complication, principal procedure) (Abdelhak, p. 79; Johns, pp. 109–110).

38.

B. To ultimately determine the DRG, first identify and code the principal diagnosis. Then the major diagnostic category can be determined. The decision tree within the Major Diagnostic Category can be consulted and the specific DRG determined. It is important to have an understanding of the manual assignment of DRGs (Abdelhak, pp. 238–239; Johns, pp. 371–372; Rogers, p. 39).

39.

B. Day outliers are cases that have exceptionally long lengths of stay. Cost outliers are cases that have reasonable lengths of stay but very high consumption of resources (Abdelhak, p. 158; Johns, p. 373).

40.

B. The UB-92, or Uniform Bill-92, was designed to reduce paperwork and errors in billing, provide faster reimbursement, and reduce training needs. Physician offices submit their Medicare claims on a different form, the HCFA-1500 (Abdelhak, p. 235; Buck, p. 386; Johns, p. 385).

41.

A. The retrospective fee-for-service reimbursement system did not encourage cost containment and in 1982, Congress determined that health care costs had reached critical dimensions. The Tax Equity and Fiscal Responsibility Act (passed in 1982, implemented in 1983) resulted in the development and implementation of a Prospective Payment System for hospitals (Abdelhak, pp. 9, 41; Johns, p. 256).

42.

B. It is the attending physician's responsibility to designate the principal diagnosis on an inpatient case. The diagnosis is coded according to ICD-9-CM and the DRG determined (Abdelhak, p. 235; Johns, pp. 370–371, 373).

43.

A. Should the facility be reimbursed more than the cost of care to the patient, as long as they have submitted proper codes, the facility can keep the surplus funds. Conversely, should the cost to care for a patient be more than the DRG rate, the facility must absorb that loss. If the case can be documented as a day or cost outlier, the facility would be eligible for additional reimbursement. Even with this additional reimbursement, however, the facility may still need to absorb some cost of the care because outlier reimbursement may be insufficient (Abdelhak, p. 158; Johns, p. 373).

44.

A. The principal procedure is one performed for therapeutic rather than diagnostic purposes, that is performed to resolve a complication, or that is most closely related to the principal diagnosis (Abdelhak, p. 87).

45.

D. The purpose of the Prospective Payment System is to set limits on Medicare spending (Abdelhak, pp. 236–238; Buck, p. 571).

46.

D. In order to calculate the conversion factor for CPT coding reimbursement, you multiple the RVUs by conversion factor (Abdelhak, p. 624; Buck, p. 576).

5 ICD-9-CM and CPT-4 Coding

objectives

After completion of this chapter, the student will be able to:

➤ Identify the formats of the ICD-9-CM and CPT-4 manual.

➤ Apply the coding conventions used in the ICD–9-CM and CPT-4 systems.

➤ Utilize the Official Guidelines for Inpatient and Outpatient Coding Guidelines in order to assign valid diagnostic and/or procedure codes.

DIRECTIONS (Questions 1–200): Each of the questions or incomplete statements below is followed by suggested answers or completions. Select the **best** answer in each case.

1. Left main coronary artery disease. Hypertension (medication was administered during the admission). Coronary bypass, left internal mammary artery to left anterior descending and saphenous vein to obtuse marginal. Temporary pacing wire inserted.
   A. 414.01, 401.9, 36.12, 39.64
   B. 414.9, 401.9, 36.12, 37.78
   C. 414.04, 401.9, 36.14, 37.78
   D. 414.00, 401.9, 36.12, 36.15, 39.64

2. Six-month-old infant with mass in right inguinal region. Indirect inguinal hernia with incarceration and ovarian cyst found during surgery. Right inguinal herniorrhaphy with placement of mesh and ovarian cystectomy.
   A. 552.9, 756.79, 53.03, 65.29
   B. 550.00, 620.8, 53.01, 65.29
   C. 550.10, 620.2, 53.04, 65.29
   D. 550.10, 620.9, 53.00, 65.29

3. Urinary incontinence due to cystocele and rectocele. Anterior and posterior colporrhaphy.
   A. 618.0, 788.30, 70.50
   B. 618.0, 70.51, 70.52
   C. 596.8, 70.51, 70.52
   D. 618.4, 625.6, 70.50

4. Calcaneus and tarsal coalition, left foot. Left subtalar fusion with tibial bone graft.
   A. 755.67, 755.69, 77.77, 81.20
   B. 755.67, 77.77, 78.00, 81.13
   C. 755.8, 78.07, 81.13
   D. 755.9, 78.48, 81.13

5. Confirmed ruptured spleen (result of car accident). Exploratory laparotomy and splenectomy.
   A. 289.59, E819, 41.43
   B. 767.8, E819.9, 41.99
   C. 865.04, E819.9, 41.5
   D. 865.09, E819, 41.5

6. Cellulitis involving right foot; some acute ascending lymphangitis visible as well. Incision and drainage; debridement of abscess on right foot.
   A. 457.2, 86.01, 86.28
   B. 682.7, 86.01, 86.28
   C. 682.7, 457.2, 86.22, 86.09
   D. 682.7, 041.10, 86.22, 86.09

7. Lumbar spinal stenosis (L4-5, L5-S1). Persistent right leg pain. Lumbar decompression of L4 to sacrum, bilateral foraminotomies of L5 and S1 bilaterally, and bilateral lateral fusion of L4 to sacrum using iliac crest bone graft.
   A. 729.5, 03.09, 81.07, 78.09
   B. 729.5, 724.09, 03.09, 81.07
   C. 724.02, 03.09, 81.07, 78.09
   D. 724.02, 03.09, 81.07

8. Symptomatic uterine prolapse, cystocele and rectocele. Vaginal hysterectomy; anterior and posterior colporrhaphy.
   A. 618.0, 68.59, 70.51, 70.52
   B. 618.1, 68.7, 70.50
   C. 618.8, 68.7, 70.51, 70.52
   D. 618.4, 68.59, 70.50

9. Postoperative sepsis, left knee. Culture revealed staphylococcus aureus. Arthroscopy; irrigation and debridement of left anterior knee joint; partial synovectomy.
   A. 682.9, 038.11, 80.76, 80.86
   B. 998.59, 038.11, 80.86, 80.76

C. 038.9, 80.26, 86.28, 80.76. 96.59

D. 998.59, 682.9, 038.11, 86.28, 80.76

10. Comminuted intertrochanteric left hip fracture. Compression hip fixation, left hip.

A. 820.21, 81.40

B. 733.14

C. 820.9

D. 820.31

11. Intertrochanteric fracture. Open reduction, right hip; pin was inserted.

A. 820.31, 79.30

B. 820.8, 79.30

C. 820.21, 79.35

D. 820.09, 79.39

12. Left thyroid nodule. Left thyroid lobectomy.

A. 193, 06.31

B. 226, 06.39

C. 239.7, 06.51

D. 241.0, 06.2

13. Pain, left lower leg. Patient fell into a hole in his backyard. X-ray revealed displaced left lower leg fracture of tibia. Open reduction and internal fixation of displaced fracture, left distal tibia; application of short leg fiberglass cast.

A. 824.80, E883.9, 79.36

B. 823.80, E883.9, E849.0, 79.06

C. 823.80, 729.5, E833.9, 79.26

D. 824.90, E833.9, 79.16

14. Dominant right shoulder impingement syndrome and right rotator cuff tear. Right shoulder examination under anesthesia; right shoulder acromioplasty and rotator cuff repair.

A. 724.4, 880.00, 89.39, 81.82

B. 726.2, 840.4, 81.83, 83.63

C. 726.19, 879.8, 81.83, 83.63

D. 726.0, 879.9, 89.39, 81.82

15. Coronary artery disease. Angioplasty showed 100% occlusion of left anterior descending artery. Aortocoronary bypass graft, left anterior descending and diagonal coronary artery; insertion of temporary pacing wire.

A. 414.01, 411.81, 36.12, 37.78

B. 414.9, 410.9, 36.11, 37.78

C. 429.2, 411.81, 36, 36.12

D. 440.8, 410.8, 36.11, 37.78

16. Left eye phacoemulsification with implantation of posterior chamber intraocular lens.

A. 66983

B. 66984

C. 66850, 66985

D. 66830

17. Excision of Morton's neuroma, right 3-4.

A. 28030

B. 64776

C. 28080

D. 64783

18. Diagnostic and surgical laparoscopy, excision of right ovarian lesion, and left oophorectomy. Diagnostic hysteroscopy, endometrial biopsy, and uterine curettage.

A. 58662, 58661, 58558

B. 58600, 58661, 58605, 58558

C. 58662, 58605, 58561

D. 58661, 58600, 58662, 58558

19. Arthroscopy. Medial meniscectomy. Debridement by shaving, cartilage of left knee.

A. 29870, 29881, 29877

B. 29881, 29877

C. 29881, 29870

D. 29881

20. Right hydrocelectomy.

A. 55000

B. 55040

C. 55041

D. 55060

21. Dr. Drew sees a patient in the emergency room complaining of abdominal pain. He provides a problem-focused history and examination, which reveals the abdominal pain beginning 2 days ago. The abdominal pain is extremely painful, with some nausea and fatigue. The patient did not take any medication for the pain. Dr. Drew orders a HCG test and urinalysis, which reveals negative HCG and UTI due to E-coli.
    A. 99281
    B. 99282
    C. 99283
    D. 99284

22. Repair of reducible right inguinal hernia with Marlex mesh. The patient is 18 years old.
    A. 49520
    B. 49505
    C. 49520, 49568
    D. 49505, 49568

23. Exploration of dorsum of left wrist with transfer of abductor pollicis longus to extensor pollicis longus.
    A. 25100, 26492
    B. 25100, 26494
    C. 25101, 26496
    D. 25101, 26494

24. Laparoscopic cholecystectomy.
    A. 47562
    B. 47600
    C. 47563
    D. 47564

25. Endometrial ablation via electrocautery, hysteroscopy.
    A. 17200, 58563
    B. 58563
    C. 58558, 58563
    D. 49200

26. Partial hymenectomy.
    A. 56720
    B. 56620
    C. 56740
    D. 56700

27. Left tympanostomy, insertion of ventilating tube. Patient received a local anesthetic.
    A. 69433
    B. 69799
    C. 69631
    D. 69436

28. Cystourethroscopy with urethral dilation.
    A. 52214
    B. 52260
    C. 52281
    D. 52290

29. Wide excision of .5 centimeter right breast lesion (carcinoma).
    A. 19120
    B. 19101
    C. 11600
    D. 11620

30. Hysteroscopy with dilation and curettage.
    A. 58558
    B. 49320, 58120
    C. 58555, 58120
    D. 49320, 57800

31. Severe diverticulitis of transverse colon. Temporary ileostomy created; resection of a portion of the transverse colon with end-to-end colostomy.
    A. 562.11, 45.74, 46.21
    B. 562.11, 45.74, 46.21, 45.94
    C. 751.5, 45.74, 46.21
    D. 562.11, 45.74, 45.94

32. Compound fractures, mandible and right superior and inferior maxilla. Open reduction

of mandible with internal fixation; open reduction of maxilla with alloplastic implant.
A. 802.9, 76.74, 76.76
B. 802.5, 802.30, 76.74, 76.76, 76.92
C. 804.5, 76.79, 76.92
D. 802.39, 76.71, 76.74, 76.92

33. Laceration of the left lung, the result of a gunshot wound. Pneumonotomy; exploration of wound area; removal of bullet from lung; closure of laceration.
A. 861.22, E985.4, 33.43, 34.02
B. 861.32, E985.4, 33.43, 33.1
C. 934.8, E985.4, 33.43, 33.99
D. 908.0, E985.4, 33.1, 33.49

34. Pregnancy at term delivered spontaneously in parking lot just prior to admission, liveborn female infant, vertex presentation. Patient examined in the delivery room; first-degree laceration repaired.
A. V24.0, V27.0, 71.71
B. 650, V27.0, 71.71
C. 664.01, V24.0, V27.0, 75.69
D. 664.04, V27.0, 75.69

35. Pregnancy at term delivered of liveborn male infant. Spontaneous ROA delivery. Poor contractions during first 8 hours of labor; intravenous Pitocin drip administered to augment labor. Episiotomy.
A. 650, V27.0, 73.6, 73.4
B. 661.11, V27.0, 73.6
C. 659.91, V27.0, 73.6, 73.4
D. 66.11, V27.0, 73.6

36. Infant weighing 2,550 grams born at 35 weeks to diabetic mother by cesarean section. Transient hypoglycemia was also documented.
A. V27.0, 775.1, 251.1
B. V30.01, 766.1, 775.6
C. 648.01, V27.0, 251.2
D. V30.01, 765.19, 775.1

37. Ruptured ectopic tubal pregnancy; acute urinary tract infection developed on second postoperative day. Left salpingo-oophorectomy.
A. 633.1, 599.0, 65.49
B. 633.10, 599.0, 66.62
C. 633.1, 639.8, 66.62, 65.39
D. 633.1, 599.0, 66.62, 65.39

38. Pregnancy at term delivered of liveborn male by low forceps and episiotomy. Delivery room record mentions cord around neck once, loose; no evidence of fetal problem.
A. 663.11, 669.51, V27.0, 72.1
B. 663.21, 669.51, V27.0, 72.1
C. 663.31, 669.51, V27.0, 72.1
D. 663.31, 669.51, 72.1

39. Pregnancy at term delivered of liveborn female, breech with obstructed labor. Total breech extraction with forceps to head.
A. 652.11, 660.01, 72.53
B. 652.21, 72.53
C. 660.01, 652.21, 72.53
D. 660.01, 72.53

40. Patient was brought to emergency room at 4:10 A.M. Patient left the emergency room against medical advice at 4:50 A.M. without being examined.
A. V64.2
B. 799.9
C. V71.9
D. E928.9

41. Conversion reaction with symptoms of chest pain and generalized weakness.
A. 786.50, 728.9, 300.11
B. 300.11, 786.50, 780.7
C. 300.11, 413.9, 428.9
D. 300.11

42. Arteriosclerotic cardiovascular disease.
    A. 429.2, 440.9
    B. 429.2
    C. 414.0, 402.90
    D. 414.0, 440.9

43. Five-hour-old infant, premature at 30 weeks, the result of a spontaneous birth, was transferred from Hospital A to the neonatal intensive care unit at Hospital B. Final diagnosis at Hospital B: male newborn, suspected respiratory distress due to prematurity.
    A. V30.00, 765.00, 73.59
    B. 765.10, 769
    C. 765.10, V71.8
    D. V30.00, 765.10, 769

44. Tumor of sacral spinal cord.
    A. 192.2
    B. 198.3
    C. 237.5
    D. 239.7

45. Live twin at term born by total breech extraction. Fractured femur, shaft, upper third. Fracture manipulation and cast. Liveborn mate was vertex and spontaneous.
    A. V31.00, 821.01, 763.1, 79.75
    B. V33.00, 754.30, 763.0, 79.75
    C. V31.00, 767.3, 763.0, 79.05
    D. V31.00, 767.3, 821.01, 763.0, 79.05, 93.53

46. Total abdominal hysterectomy, bilateral salpingo-oophorectomy. Incidental appendectomy. Culdoplasty.
    A. 58150, 44955, 58999
    B. 58150, 56800
    C. 58200, 44950
    D. 58150, 44955

47. Uvulopalatopharyngoplasty (laser assisted).
    A. 42145
    B. 42205

C. 42180
D. 42200

48. Evacuation of subdural hematoma.
    A. 61314
    B. 61108
    C. 61313
    D. 61312

49. Second-look exploratory laparotomy along with jejunoileostomy. History of colon cancer.
    A. 58960, 44310
    B. 49008, 44300
    C. 49000, 44310
    D. 58960

50. Left extracorporeal shock wave lithotripsy, left kidney.
    A. 33960, 50590
    B. 50590
    C. 33961, 50590
    D. 52337

51. Closed reduction and cannulated screw fixation of left Lisfranc's dislocation/fracture (one bone). Application of short leg cast.
    A. 28470
    B. 28475
    C. 28476
    D. 28485

52. Right carotid endarterectomy.
    A. 60600
    B. 33572
    C. 35390
    D. 35301

53. Dr. Sienta provides critical care services in the ER for 45-year-old patient who was involved in an altercation. The patient has a closed head injury with a subdural hemorrhage. In addition, the patient is in respira-

tory failure. Total critical care 1½ hours for this patient.

A. 99291 × 1

B. 99292 × 1 AND 99292 × 1

C. 99291 × 1 AND 99292 × 2

D. 99291 × 1 AND 99292 × 3

54. Right carpal tunnel release.

A. 64721

B. 64722

C. 25020

D. 25023

55. Small bowel resection.

A. 44120

B. 49000, 44130

C. 44120

D. 44130

56. Laparoscopic cholecystectomy.

A. 47560

B. 47562

C. 47600

D. 47610

57. Subsequent hospital visit for a 73-year-old female with severe COPD and broncho-spasm; initially admitted for acute respira-tory distress requiring ventilatory support in the ICU. The patient was stabilized, extu-bated, and transferred to the floor, but has now developed acute fever, dyspnea, left lower lobe rhonchi, and laboratory evidence of carbon dioxide retention and hypoxemia.

A. 99231

B. 99232

C. 99233

D. 99223

58. Esophagogastroduodenoscopy with open Stamm gastrostomy tube.

A. 43219

B. 43235

C. 43246

D. 44372

59. Oral rehabilitation; preparation of maxillary right quadrant for dentures via alveolo-plasty.

A. 92510

B. 41872

C. 92526, 21089

D. 41874

60. Repair of incarcerated umbilical hernia with omental resection.

A. 49587, 49255

B. 49585, 49999

C. 49585, 49905

D. 49587

61. Bronchopneumonia due to *Diplococcus pneumoniae;* diabetes mellitus. The patient was on insulin during admission; discharge instructions included daily insulin injections.

A. 481, 250.01

B. 485, 041.2, 250.01

C. 481, 250.00

D. 485, 041.2, 250.91

62. Acute pulmonary edema due to inhalation of chlorine fumes. Patient works at a chemi-cal plant where transport pipes burst, caus-ing contact.

A. 506.1, E869.8

B. 987.6, 506.1, E869.8

C. 518.4, E869.8, E849.3

D. 987.6, 508.8, E982.8

63. Diabetic intercapillary glomerulosclerosis and peripheral angiopathy. For the past 5 years, the patient has been on daily insulin injections.

A. 250.81, 581.81, 443.81

B. 250.40, 250.70, 581.81, 443.81

C. 581.81, 443.81, 250.40, 250.70

D. 250.41, 250.71, 581.81, 443.81

64. Diabetes mellitus due to long-standing cortisone therapy for psoriatic arthritis.
    A. 250.00, 696.0, E932.0
    B. 962.0, 250.00, 696.0, E932.0
    C. 250.01, 696.0, E932.0
    D. 251.8, 696.0, E932.0

65. Uncontrolled insulin-dependent diabetes mellitus.
    A. 250.01
    B. 250.91
    C. 250.03
    D. 250.93

66. Fibroma, left forearm, with evidence of invasive activity.
    A. 171.2
    B. 215.2
    C. 238.1
    D. 195.4

67. Carcinoma of the right lung with liver metastasis. Status post right pneumonectomy 2 years ago. Patient underwent chemotherapy during this admission.
    A. V58.1, 197.7, V10.11, 99.25
    B. 162.9, 197.7, V58.1, 99.25
    C. V58.1, 197.7, V45.89, 99.25
    D. 162.9, 197.7, V45.89, 99.25

68. Carcinoma of the peritoneum, primary site undetermined.
    A. 197.6, 158.9
    B. 239.0, 199.1
    C. 158.9, 199.1
    D. 197.6, 199.1

69. Epidermoid carcinoma of the leg.
    A. 195.5
    B. 173.7
    C. 239.8
    D. 706.2

70. Patient had carcinoma of anterior bladder wall fulgurated 3 years ago. The patient returns annually for recheck cystoscopy. Patient is currently admitted for a routine recheck. A small recurring malignancy is found and fulgurated during cystoscopy.
    A. 188.3, 57.32
    B. V67.9, V10.51, 57.49
    C. V67.0, V10.51, 57.49, 57.32
    D. 188.3, 57.49

71. Choriocarcinoma of the corpus uteri with metastasis to pelvic lymph nodes. Total hysterectomy; biopsy of suspicious lymph node. Chemotherapy is administered for metastasis. Patient has severe residuals to chemotherapy.
    A. 182.0, 196.6, V58.1, 995.2, E933.1, 68.4, 40.11, 99.25
    B. 182.0, 198.82, V58.1, 909.9, E933.1, 68.4, 40.11, 99.25
    C. 182.0, 196.6, V58.1, 995.2, E933.1, 64.8, 40.11, 99.25
    D. V58.1, 182.0, V10.3, 963.1, E980.4, 68.4, 68.13, 99.25

72. Patient is being treated by his personal physician with Valium. Today at lunch he had three whiskey sours. By 5:00 P.M., the patient was unconscious.
    A. 780.00, 980.0, 964.4, E939.4, E947.8
    B. 780.09, E939.4, E947.8, E980.3
    C. 969.4, 980.0, 780.09, E853.2, E860.0
    D. 969.4, 780.4, E947.8, E860.0, E980.3

73. Patient has a history of thrombophlebitis of the leg and is taking Coumadin. Three days ago she fell and sustained a severe bruise to the left shoulder. Because of pain, she took 10 g aspirin q4h. After 3 days of aspirin therapy, patient is admitted for severe abdominal pain, which proves to be internal

hemorrhage as an adverse effect of the drug combination.

A. 964.2, 965.1, 459.0, E858.2, E850.3
B. 459.0, 909.0, V12.5, E929.2
C. 964.2, 965.1, 958.2, E858.2, E850.3
D. 459.0, 451.2, E934.2, E935.3

74. Patient complains of extreme dizziness and weakness; admission diagnosis is possible cerebrovascular accident. Study shows that symptoms are an adverse effect of Isordil (isosorbide dinitrate). Patient is on 5 milligrams Isordil 3 times a day for angina, as prescribed by her physician.

A. 413.9, 780.4, 780.7, E942.4
B. 436, 972.4, 780.4, 780.7, E858.3
C. 972.4, 780.4, 780.7, 413.9, E858.3
D. 780.4, 780.7, 413.9, E942.4

75. Patient takes Eskalith, 450 milligrams b.i.d. and is seen weekly at the clinic. Patient's record was lost and patient was seen in the hypertension clinic where Aldomet was ordered. Patient did not reveal taking any other medication, although Eskalith and Aldomet are contraindicated. Patient admitted for seizures due to lithium intoxication.

A. 780.39, E939.8, E942.6
B. 780.39, V71.8, E939.8, E942.6
C. 969.8, 972.6, 780.39, E855.8, E858.3
D. 780.39, 969.8, 972.6, E855.8, E858.3

76. Split thickness skin graft from left thigh to axilla, 25 square centimeter area.

A. 15100
B. 14021
C. 15120
D. 15000, 15100

77. Feeding jejunostomy.

A. 44799
B. 44015
C. 44310
D. 48001

78. Right pterional craniotomy for electrothrombosis of intracranial middle cerebral artery aneurysm.

A. 61556, 61700
B. 61708
C. 61556, 61708
D. 61705

79. Modified radical mastectomy with free transverse rectus abdominis myocutaneous flap reconstruction.

A. 19240, 19364
B. 19200, 19367
C. 19240, 19367
D. 19220, 19364

80. Free rectus abdominis free flap to right foot. Soleus turnover rotation flat to right foot, 10 square centimeters. Split thickness skin graft, 200 square centimeters to right lower leg. Amputation of right great toe at metatarsal level. Debridement of skin and subcutaneous tissue.

A. 15100, 15101, 28810, 11042
B. 15738, 14040, 15100, 15101, 28810
C. 15738, 15101, 28810, 11040
D. 15756, 15100, 15101, 28820, 11041

81. Repeat low transverse cesarean section.

A. 59620
B. 59612
C. 59514
D. 59618

82. Resection of brain tumor, posterior fossa.

A. 61526
B. 61518
C. 61510
D. 61545

83. Diagnostic and operative laparoscopy with biopsy.
    A. 49321
    B. 47561
    C. 49321, 49320
    D. 58662

84. Appendectomy.
    A. 44950
    B. 44955
    C. 44960
    D. 44900

85. Excision of ganglion, right index finger.
    A. 25111
    B. 25112
    C. 26160
    D. 11420

86. Excision of 5-centimeter malignant lesion of the right supraclavicular area.
    A. 11406
    B. 11400
    C. 11600
    D. 11606

87. Excision of 3.5-centimeter squamous cell carcinoma, right side of face; wound closure with 4 sutures of interrupted 5:0 prolene.
    A. 11604
    B. 11624
    C. 11404
    D. 11644

88. Fracture of the left humerus. Patient transferred for definitive care. Long arm cast applied for patient comfort during transport.
    A. 99070
    B. 29065
    C. 24500
    D. 24516

89. Sigmoidoscopy.
    A. 45332
    B. 45330
    C. 45355
    D. 45334

90. Excision of a 3 × 2 cm basal cell carcinoma of the left side of the forehead.
    A. 11643
    B. 11603
    C. 11623
    D. 11646

91. Hypertensive cardiovascular disease with congestive heart failure; benign essential hypertension.
    A. 402.11, 401.1
    B. 428.0, 429, 440.9
    C. 401.1, 428.0, 429.2
    D. 402.11

92. Uremia; cardiomegaly; malignant hypertension.
    A. 586, 429.3, 401.1
    B. 404.00
    C. 405.01, 429.3
    D. 403.00, 429.3

93. Hemiplegia secondary to cerebral artery thrombosis 8 months ago.
    A. 342.9, 436
    B. 434.0, 342.9
    C. 342.9, 438
    D. 433.9, 342.9

94. Angina; permanent cardiac pacemaker inserted 1 year ago, functioning well.
    A. 413.9, V45.01
    B. 428.9, V53.3
    C. 413.9, V42.2
    D. 413.9, V43.3

95. Sipple's syndrome with hypertension.
    A. 193, 401.0
    B. 193, 401.9
    C. 193, 405.09
    D. 193, 405.99

96. Scars of face from third-degree burns sustained in house fire at 9 months of age. Revision of scars by Z-plasty and excision of scar tissue.
    A. 941.30, 709.2, E929.4, 86.84
    B. 709.2, 906.5, E929.4, 86.3
    C. 709.2, 906.5, E890.9, 86.3
    D. 941.30, 709.2, E890.9, 86.84

97. Post-concussion brain syndrome following auto collision with another motor vehicle on a public highway. No loss of consciousness. Patient admitted for evaluation.
    A. 310.2, E815.9
    B. 310.2, 850.0, E815.9
    C. 850.0, E815.9
    D. 310.2, 907.0, E929.0

98. Missile fracture of tibial shaft, upper section.
    A. 823.20
    B. 823.30
    C. 823.00, 823.20
    D. 823.10

99. Pathological fracture of the intertrochanteric section, left femur. Osteoporosis, generalized, postmenopausal.
    A. 820.31, 733.01
    B. 820.21, 733.01
    C. 733.14, 733.01
    D. 733.15, 733.00

100. Third-degree burns, left arm and chest. Second- and third-degree burns on the abdomen and left leg. Fifty percent of body surface is burned, 20% are third-degree burns.
    A. 942.30, 943.30, 945.30, 945.20, 948.52
    B. 942.39, 943.30, 945.20, 945.30, 948.52
    C. 942.30, 943.30, 945.20, 948.25, 948.52
    D. 942.32, 942.33, 943.30, 945.30, 948.52

101. Infected second-degree burns of the hand from boiling water.
    A. 906.6, 958.3, E924.0
    B. 958.3, 944.20, E924.0
    C. 958.3, 906.6, E929.8
    D. 944.20, 958.3, E924.0

102. A 50-year-old woman had a suprapubic bladder tube inserted 2 days ago and is now admitted with gross hematuria with clots. A cystoscopy and evacuation of clots was performed.
    A. 996.76, 57.32, 57.0
    B. 996.70, 57.93
    C. 599.7, 57.32, 57.0
    D. 596.7, 57.93

103. Male patient admitted with exacerbation of his multiple sclerosis. He feels weak as a result. Patient is paraplegic as a result of the multiple sclerosis.
    A. 780.7, 340
    B. 340, 780.7
    C. 780.7, 344.1
    D. 340, 344.1

104. Acute gangrenous appendicitis. Postoperative paralytic ileus. Appendectomy.
    A. 540.9, 560.1, 47.09
    B. 540.9, 564.4, 47.09
    C. 540.0, 560.9, 47.09
    D. 540.9, 997.4, 47.09

105. Peritonitis due to catheter inserted into abdomen for ambulatory peritoneal dialysis. Removal of catheter.
   A. 996.62, 97.82
   B. 567.8, 97.82
   C. 998.5, 97.82
   D. 996.1, 97.82

106. Excision of 1.5 cm face lesion (Bowenoid Senile Keratosis).
   A. 11443
   B. 11442
   C. 11643
   D. 11642

107. Excision of 1 cm and 2 × 1 cm benign forehead lesions, on the right.
   A. 11424
   B. 11443, 11441
   C. 11423
   D. 11442, 11441

108. Needle biopsy, bone marrow.
   A. 85095
   B. 38230
   C. 38221
   D. 85097

109. Excision of 2 × 1 × 1 cm malignant metastatic lesion of the right supraclavicular area.
   A. 11601
   B. 11602
   C. 11603
   D. 11604

110. Cholecystectomy; incidental appendectomy.
   A. 47600
   B. 47600, 44950
   C. 56340, 44950
   D. 56342

111. Angioplasty of right coronary artery.
   A. 92984
   B. 35452
   C. 92986
   D. 92982

112. Biopsy of endometrium.
   A. 58100
   B. 56351
   C. 56305
   D. 57500

113. Total abdominal hysterectomy and bilateral salpingo-oophorectomy.
   A. 58262
   B. 58200
   C. 58152
   D. 58150

114. Reduction and skeletal traction, right open tibial shaft fracture.
   A. 27532
   B. 27752
   C. 27762
   D. 27825

115. Reduction of open wrist fracture and 2 cm wound closure.
   A. 25680
   B. 25685, 12001
   C. 25680, 12001
   D. 25685

116. Bilateral oophorectomy by laparoscopy for benign ovarian cyst.
   A. 58661
   B. 58262
   C. 58940
   D. 58720

117. Primary low transverse cesarean section for twin gestation.
    A. 59620
    B. 59610
    C. 59514
    D. 59612

118. Coronary artery bypass graft of 2 vessels.
    A. 33534
    B. 33511
    C. 33533
    D. 33518

119. Laparoscopically assisted vaginal hysterectomy, bilateral salpingo-oophorectomy.
    A. 56301, 58263
    B. 56301, 56308
    C. 56301, 58260, 58263
    D. 58550

120. Intravenous infusion chemotherapy × 3 hours.
    A. 96408, 96410, 96412, 96545
    B. 96410, 96412, 96412, 96545
    C. 96408, 96412, 96545
    D. 96410, 96412, 96412

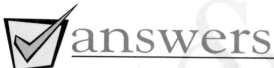

answers & rationales

1.

A. Assign two separate codes for the left main coronary artery disease and hypertension because no cause-and-effect relationship regarding the hypertension and heart disease was stated. If there is no mention in the health record of the patient having undergone a bypass code 414.01, arteriosclerosis of native coronary artery should be assigned. Patient underwent coronary bypass of two vessels (left internal mammary to left anterior descending and saphenous vein to obtuse marginal). In addition, a temporary pacing wire was inserted during the bypass procedure (Brown, pp. 257–258, 266, 272, 277).

2.

C. The term incarcerated refers to "with obstruction." The diagnosis in this question would be "unilateral indirect inguinal hernia with obstruction." Also assign a code for ovarian cyst. For the hernia procedure, mesh is used to reinforce the hernia repair and is considered a prosthesis or graft (Brown, pp. 161–162).

3.

A. Cystocele and rectocele are classified using the same ICD-9-CM code number. The urinary incontinence is also coded because of the instruction, "Use additional code to identify urinary incontinence . . ." located below category 618. Stress incontinence is not stated in the question; therefore, assign 788.30 for symptomatic incontinence. A combination code is assigned to classify the anterior and posterior repair procedure (Brown, p. 171).

4.

B. Subclassification code 755.67 includes the following congenital anomalies: calcaneus and tarsal coalition. Note the "code also" instruction located under subcategory 78.0; a code needs to be assigned to classify the excision of bone for grafting purposes. It is also important to note that there is no statement as to the site of the bone excision for the graft (Brown, pp. 193–202).

5.

C. Review all terms below the subterm entry in ICD-9-CM Volume 2; in this question, the splenic rupture was traumatic. In addition, the Index to External Causes must also be referenced to classify the cause of the trauma (motor vehicle accident). The fourth-digit subcategories are listed below the title, "Motor Vehicle Traffic Accidents (E810-E819)," in ICD-9-CM Volume 1. The splenectomy is coded as total because code 41.5 includes "splenectomy NOS." Do not assign a code to the exploratory laparotomy because a definitive procedure was performed during the surgery. Note the instruction located below the index reference for laparotomy; it states that when the laparotomy is performed "as operative approach C omit code" (Brown, pp. 50, 308–310).

6.

B. It is not necessary to assign a code to the acute ascending lymphangitis; refer to the "includes" note under category 682. Note that the debridement was not stated as excisional type (Brown, pp. 73–75, 188).

7.

D. Right leg pain is a symptom of the lumbar spinal stenosis and would not be assigned a code. In this question, the lumbar decompression of L4 to sacrum was not considered exploratory and would be coded. The "includes" note under subcategory 81.0 states "arthrodesis of spine with: bone graft. . . ." Therefore, it is not necessary to assign a separate code to the iliac crest bone graft (Brown, pp. 73–75, 47–58).

8.

D. A combination code is assigned to classify the uterine prolapse, cystocele and rectocele, as well as the anterior and posterior colporrhaphy. The vaginal hysterectomy is classified as "other" because it was not stated as "radical" (Brown, p. 171, Buck, p. 116).

9.

B. The sepsis in the patient's left knee is considered a complication of the incision and drainage procedure performed previously. A code is also assigned to the staphylococcus aureus per the instruction, "Use additional code to identify infection," located under code 998.59. An irrigation and debridement was performed via arthroscopy; the debridement was not of skin but of the joint and is to be coded accordingly. Because this is a debridement of the knee joint, the coder is instructed to see "Excision, lesion, joint." The coder should also separately code the synovectomy (Brown, pp. 344–345).

10.

A. The comminuted intertrochanteric fracture is not stated as opened or closed; therefore, code it as closed. The compression hip fixation does not specify whether an external or internal device was utilized. Therefore, when the coder references the term, fixation, (s)he will next reference the subterm, hip. When verifying code 81.40, note that this is a "not elsewhere classified" code assignment (Brown, p. 313).

11.

C. In the ICD-9-CM index, Fracture, intertrochanteric, instructs the coder to see Fracture, femur, neck, in-

tertrochanteric. The fact that an open repair was performed does not indicate an open fracture; therefore, assign the code to indicate a closed fracture. When coding the procedure, refer to Reduction, fracture, femur, open, with internal fixation and verify code 79.35 in the tabular. The pin is the internal fixation device and is not coded separately (Brown, pp. 313–315).

12.

D. When coding a lesion, refer to the ICD-9-CM Volume 2 main term for the type of lesion or growth, instead of first referencing the Neoplasm Table. In this question, the main term, nodule, is listed in the alphabetical index; by going to the Neoplasm Table, an incorrect code assignment would result. To code the thyroid lobectomy, refer to lobectomy in Volume 3 of ICD-9-CM and verify code 06.2 in the tabular. Referencing the main term, excision, and subterms, lesion, thyroid, results in an incorrect code assignment (Brown, pp. 287–288).

13.

A. Although the x-ray impression did not state that the fracture was of the distal tibia, the operative procedure indicates the location of the fracture. According to Brown, "further review of the health record is needed to ensure complete and accurate coding." In addition, the fracture is not stated as opened or closed; therefore, code it as closed. The pain in the left lower leg would not be coded because this is a symptom of the fracture. Be sure to assign the E code to indicate the external cause of the fracture and the place it occurred. To code the repair, reference the main term, reduction, in Volume 3 of ICD-9-CM and subterms, tibia, open, with internal fixation; verify code 79.36 in the tabular. Do not code the application of a short leg fiberglass cast; the index instructs the coder to see Reduction, fracture when the cast application is performed with a fracture reduction (Brown, pp. 313–318).

14.

B. It is necessary to assign multiple codes as needed. This coding guideline is applied in this question by assigning more than one code to the conditions and procedures stated (Brown, p. 37).

15.

A. Referencing disease, coronary artery in Volume 2 of ICD-9-CM instructs the coder to see Arteriosclerosis, coronary. After following this instruction, the coder should then verify code 414.00 in the tabular. The occluded vessel noted during angiogram should be coded by referencing the main term, occlusion, and subterms, artery, coronary, without myocardial infarction. Verify code 411.81 in the tabular. The patient underwent aortocoronary bypass of two coronary arteries (left anterior descending coronary artery and diagonal coronary artery). In addition, a temporary pacing wire was inserted during the procedure (Brown, pp. 257–258, 266, 272, 277).

16.

B. Phacoemulsification requires the use of an ultrasonic device to disintegrate the cataract, which is then aspirated and removed. Refer to Phacoemulsification in the CPT index and review codes 66982 and 66984. Code 66984 describes extracapsular cataract extraction with insertion of intraocular lens prosthesis (CPT, pp. 206, 487).

17.

C. Morton's neuroma is a neuroma-like mass of the neurovascular bundle of the intermetatarsal spaces. Intermetatarsal spaces refer to the region of the foot that contains the five metatarsal bones. A Morton's neuroma located on the right, between the third and fourth metatarsal bones, would be described as Morton's neuroma, right 3-4. Code 28080 describes an excision of one interdigital (Morton's) neuroma. Refer to index Morton's neuroma excision, see code 28080 (CPT, pp. 95, 472).

18.

A. The diagnostic laparoscopy is included with the code for a surgical laparoscopy. A combination code for the diagnostic and operative laparoscopy, and excision of the right ovarian lesion is assigned code 58662. The left oophorectomy is code 58661 because it was performed via laparoscopy. The diagnostic hysteroscopy with endometrial biopsy and curettage of uterus is given combination code 58558 (CPT, pp. 179–180).

19.

D. In the CPT index, refer to Arthroscopy, surgical, knee and codes 29871 to 29889. Review the range of codes on page 101 and note that code 29881 describes Arthroscopy, knee, surgical; with meniscectomy (medial OR lateral, including any meniscal shaving). A separate code for the debridement by shaving, cartilage of left knee is not assigned because the meniscus of the knee is the knee's cartilage (CPT, pp. 101, 378).

20.

B. A hydrocelectomy is the excision of a hydrocele, which is the accumulation of serous fluid in a saclike cavity, especially in the tunica vaginalis testis. Code 55040 specifically describes Excision of hydrocele; unilateral (CPT, p. 171).

21.

A. A problem-focused history; a problem-focused examination and straightforward medical decision making fall under 99281 (CPT, p. 17).

22.

B. Refer to CPT index entry, hernia, repair, inguinal, and review codes 49491, 49495 to 49500, 49505. Assign only code 49505 because according to the note located below the heading, "With the exception of the incisional hernia repairs . . . the use of mesh . . . is not separately reported." Therefore, code 49568 is not needed (CPT, pp. 156, 443).

23.

D. Refer to Exploration, wrist in the CPT index and review the listed codes. Code 25101 is selected because it describes the wrist exploration. The terms abductor pollicis longus and extensor pollicis longus refer to thumb muscles. Refer to CPT index entry, Thumb, Repair, Muscle Transfer and code number 26494, which is described as "Opponensplasty; hypothenar muscle transfer." Opponensplasty is a combining form, which means repair of muscles of the hand; hypothenar is a term that refers to the fleshy mass at the medial side of the palm (CPT, pp. 79, 84, 426, 524).

24.

A. Refer to CPT index entry, Laparoscopy, Cholecystectomy, and review codes 47562–47564. Code 47562 is described as "Laparoscopy, surgical; cholecystectomy" (CPT, p. 153, 460).

25.

B. Refer to Endometrial Ablation, Exploration via Hysteroscopy in the CPT index and review code 58563 (CPT, p. 179).

26.

D. Refer to CPT index entry, Hymenectomy and review code 56700 (CPT, p. 175).

27.

A. Refer to Insertion, Ventilating Tube in the CPT index and review code 69433. Code 69433 is described as Tympanostomy (requiring insertion of ventilating tube), local or topical anesthesia (CPT, p. 214).

28.

C. Refer to Cystourethroscopy, Dilation, Urethra in the CPT index and review code 52281 (Cystourethroscopy, with calibration and/or dilation of urethral stricture or stenosis . . .) (CPT, p. 165).

29.

A. Refer to CPT index entry, Excision, Breast, Lesion codes 19120 to 19126. Code 19120 states, "Excision of . . . malignant tumor aberrant breast tissue, . . . male or female, one or more lesions" (CPT, p. 58).

30.

A. Refer to CPT index entry, Dilation and Curettage, Hysteroscopy and review code 58558, which is described as "Hysteroscopy, surgical; . . . with or without D&C" (CPT, p. 179).

31.

A. The instruction listed below code 45.7 states to "code also any synchronous anastomosis *other than end-to-end*" (Buck, Vol. 3, p. 1069).

32.

B. Each fracture site is coded separately as no combination code exists for both sites. In addition, assign a separate code for the alloplastic implant (Buck, Vol. 1, p. 803; Vol. 3, p. 1094).

33.

B. Penetration of a bullet into the lung would puncture the lung tissue; in this question, the result was laceration of the lung tissue. The removal of the bullet from the lung is included in code 33.1 (Brown, p. 321; Buck, Vol. 1, p. 813; Vol. 3, p. 1051).

34.

D. When a patient delivers outside the hospital and is admitted for treatment of a complication, assign the code for the complication and use fifth digit *4* (Brown, p. 210).

35.

B. Poor contractions are an abnormality of labor and would therefore require this question to be coded using 661.21, not 650 (Brown, pp. 208–209).

36.

D. This infant is premature by gestational age (less than 37 weeks). Fifth digit *1* is added to indicate birth by cesarean section. Code 775.1 is assigned after referring to the exclusion note under 775.6 because the baby's mother is diabetic (Buck, Vol. 1, p. 778).

37.

C. Two codes are assigned to indicate the ectopic pregnancy and its complication. The complication is assigned a code from the 639 category. The left salpingo-oophorectomy is also assigned two codes, one to denote the salpingectomy with removal of tubal pregnancy, 66.62. The instruction below that code tells the coder to "Code also any synchronous oophorectomy." Therefore, assign code 65.39 to classify the oophorectomy (Brown, p. 223; Buck, Vol. 3, p. 1087).

38.

C. No mention is made of cord compression; therefore, 663.1 and 663.2 would be incorrect code assignments (Buck, Vol. 1, p. 741).

39.

C. The coder is instructed to "Code first any associated obstructed labor (660.0)" when referencing category code 652 (Brown, p. 209; Buck, Vol. 1, p. 741).

40.

A. When procedures are not carried out, for any reason, the code to use is V64, with an appropriate subcategory code to indicate the reason (Brown, p. 55; Buck, Vol. 1, p. 853).

41.

B. The diagnosis code is sequenced first, followed by the symptom codes. In this question, the symptoms of chest pain and generalized weakness are not integral to the conversion reaction (Brown, pp. 74–75).

42.

A. Code 429.2 instructs the coder to "Use additional code to identify presence of arteriosclerosis"; therefore, assign code 440.9 as well (Buck, Vol. 1, p. 678).

43.

B. The infant was not born at Hospital B; therefore, code V30 cannot be assigned. It would be appropriate to code both confirmed and suspected conditions during the admission at Hospital B (Brown, pp. 239–240).

44.

D. The type of tumor is not specified in this diagnostic statement; therefore, it is considered a Neoplasm of Unspecified Nature (Brown, p. 286).

45.

C. This infant was a twin with a liveborn mate; therefore, assign code V31. A fracture occurring at birth is coded to 767, not the 800 injury codes. No code is needed for application of a cast when it accompanies a reduction (Brown, pp. 239–240; Buck, Vol. 3, p. 1096).

46.

B. Refer to Hysterectomy, Abdominal, Total in the CPT index and review codes 58150 and 58200. Code 58150 describes a "Total abdominal hysterectomy (corpus and cervix), with or without removal of tube(s), with or without removal of ovary(s)." Refer to Appendectomy in the CPT index and review codes 44950 to 44960. See the note in parentheses below code 44950 that says that an "incidental appendectomy during intra-abdominal surgery does not usually warrant a separate identification." Culdoplasty is defined as "plastic surgery to remedy relaxation of the posterior fornix of the vagina." Refer to Vagina, Repair in the CPT index. Review code 56800 and note that it states, "plastic repair of introitus" (CPT, pp. 176, 375, 446, 536; Stedman's, p. 377).

47.

A. Uvulopalatopharyngoplasty (laser assisted) means "plastic surgery of the oropharynx in which redundant soft palate, uvula, pillars, fauces, and sometimes posterior pharyngeal wall mucosa are removed; the procedure may be done by using laser therapy." Because removal of tissue is stated in the definition, refer to the entry Excision, Uvula in the CPT index and review codes 42140 and 42145. Code 42145 includes the procedure, Uvulopalatopharyngoplasty, as an example (CPT, pp. 137, 425; Taber's, p. 2049).

48.

D. Refer to Hematoma, Brain, Evacuation and review codes 61312 to 61315. Code 61312 states, "Craniectomy or craniotomy for evacuation of hematoma, . . . subdural" (CPT, pp. 187, 441).

49.

C. Refer to Ileostomy in the CPT index and review codes 44310 and 45136. Its description is "Ileostomy or jejunostomy. . . ." CPT index entry Laparotomy, Second Look refers to "ovarian malignancy." Therefore, refer to Laparotomy, Exploration in the CPT index and review codes 47015, 49000 to 49002, and 58960. Code 49000 states, "Exploratory laparotomy . . ." (CPT, pp. 154, 461).

50.

B. Refer to Lithotripsy, Kidney in the CPT index and review code 50590. It states, "Lithotripsy, extracorporeal shock wave" (CPT, pp. 161, 464).

51.

C. Lisfranc's dislocation and fracture is a "dislocation of the tarsometatarsal joints of the foot by direct or indirect mechanisms; accompanying fracture is common." Refer to Fracture, Metatarsal, Closed Treatment, with Manipulation in the CPT index and review codes 28475 and 28476. Code 28476 states, "Percutaneous skeletal fixation of metatarsal fracture, with manipulation, each." The cannulated screw is a form of "percutaneous skeletal fixation"; the term reduction in the question means "manipulation," according to CPT; the term each in the code description indicates that this code is assigned once because one metatarsal fracture was treated. No code would be assigned for the cast application because the Musculoskeletal System ". . . services listed below include the application . . . of the first cast. . . ." Cast application would apply only ". . .

when the cast application . . . is a replacement procedure . . ." (CPT, pp. 97, 433; Taber's, p. 1120).

52.

D. An endarterectomy involves "excision of . . . occluding atheromatous deposits." A "thrombus . . . may be occlusive. . . ." In the CPT index, refer to Thromboendarterectomy and carotid artery and review codes 35301 and 35390. Code 35301 states, "Thromboendarterectomy, . . . carotid . . ." (CPT, pp. 122, 524; Stedman's, pp. 509, 1597).

53.

B. Refer to the Total Duration of Critical Care Table in the CPT manual (CPT, p. 20).

54.

A. Carpal Tunnel Syndrome ". . . affects some part of the median nerve distribution of the hand. . . ." CPT defines neuroplasty as "the decompression or freeing of intact nerve. . . ." Refer to Carpal Tunnel Syndrome, Decompression in the CPT index and review code 64721, which states, "Neuroplasty and/or transposition; median nerve at carpal tunnel" (CPT, pp. 200, 392; Taber's, p. 323).

55.

C. The term resection means partial excision. Refer to Intestines, Small, Excision in the CPT index and review codes 44120 to 44128. Code 44120 includes, in its description, ". . . resection of small intestine . . ." (CPT, pp. 144, 456; Taber's, p. 1659).

56.

B. Refer to Laparoscopy, Cholecystectomy in the CPT index and review codes 47562 to 47564. Code 47562 states, "Laparoscopy, surgical; cholecystectomy" (CPT, pp. 153, 460).

57.

C. Refer to E/M Section, Hospital Inpatient Services, Subsequent Hospital Care and Appendix C for case scenarios (CPT pp. 12, 350).

58.

C. Refer to Endoscopy, Gastrointestinal, Upper, Tube Placement and review code 43246. It states, "Upper gastrointestinal endoscopy, including esophagus, stomach and either the duodenum . . .; with directed placement of percutaneous gastrostomy tube" (CPT, pp. 140, 417).

59.

D. Refer to Alveoloplasty and review code 41874; it is described as "Alveoloplasty, each quadrant." Alveoloplasty is the "surgical preparation of the alveolar ridges for the reception of dentures . . ." (CPT, pp. 137, 368; Stedman's, p. 52).

60.

D. Refer to Hernia, Repair, Umbilicus, Incarcerated in the CPT index and review codes 49582 and 49587. Code 49587 states "Repair, umbilical hernia, age 5 years or over; incarcerated. . . ." For omental resection, refer to CPT index entry Excision, Omentum and when reviewing code 49255, note the phrase "(separate procedure)." The Separate Procedure explanation in CPT states, ". . . when a procedure that is ordinarily a component of a larger procedure is performed alone for a specific purpose, it may be considered a separate procedure." The omental resection was performed as part of the hernia repair procedure and would, therefore, not be assigned a separate code (CPT, pp. 156, 423, 443).

61.

A. The main term, bronchopneumonia, instructs the coder to see "Pneumonia, broncho-." Upon referencing, Pneumonia, broncho-, note that there is an additional subterm, diplococcal, indicating a code assignment of combination code 481. The patient is discharged on insulin and is, therefore, insulin dependent (Brown, p. 139; Buck, Vol. 2, p. 363).

62.

B. Cases involving poisonings require that the poisoning code be sequenced as the principal code, followed by the manifestation code, and finally the external cause (Brown, p. 335).

63.

D. Codes 250.41 and 250.71 are sequenced before codes enclosed in italics in the ICD-9-CM index. The patient is insulin dependent; therefore, fifth digit *1* will be used with these diabetes codes (Brown, pp. 93–95; Buck, Vol. 2, pp. 139–140).

64.

D. Diabetes mellitus due to a long-standing steroid (e.g., cortisone) medication administered for another condition is considered secondary diabetes and is assigned code 251.8. The development of this type of diabetes is the result of an adverse reaction to the medication administration. It would not be considered a poisoning. In the ICD-9-CM index, reference the main term, Diabetes, diabetic, and subterms, steroid induced, correct substance properly administered. It is also necessary to assign an external cause code from the ICD-9-CM Table of Drugs and Chemicals, Therapeutic Use column (E932.0). It would also be appropriate to assign a code to the psoriatic arthritis (Brown, pp. 93–95; Buck, Vol. 2, pp. 139–140, 483).

65.

C. The fourth digit subcategory for diabetes indicates the "presence of any associated complication," and the fifth-digit subclassification indicates the type of diabetes and whether it is considered out of control (or uncontrolled) (Brown, pp. 93–95).

66.

C. In the ICD-9-CM Index to Diseases, the main term Fibroma and subterm invasive instructs the coder to see Neoplasm, connective tissue, uncertain behavior. This refers the coder to the Neoplasm table in the ICD-9-CM Index to Diseases. The coder would reference Neoplasm, connective tissue, forearm, uncertain behavior and assign code 238.1 (Buck, Vol. 2, pp. 193, 311).

67.

A. Sequence the chemotherapy code first if this is the reason for admission, followed by the site of the present cancer, and then a code for history of tumor previously removed (Brown, pp. 299–300).

68.

D. When the primary site is not known, the coder must still assign a code to specify the unknown primary site (Brown, p. 292).

69.

B. In the ICD-9-CM index, the main term Carcinoma instructs the coder to see also Neoplasm, by site, malignant. The phrase epidermoid of the leg refers to skin of the leg. Therefore, the coder would refer to the Neoplasm table, skin, leg, malignant, primary and assign code 173.7 (Buck, pp. 86, 328; Stedman's, p. 522)

70.

D. A recurrent cancer at the same site is coded as a new primary. The endoscopy (i.e., cystoscopy) is included as part of code 57.49 (i.e., fulguration of recurring malignancy of bladder) (Brown, p. 300; Buck, Vol. 3, p. 1081).

71.

A. The uterine cancer is primary; the metastasis to pelvic lymph nodes is secondary. The severe residuals to chemotherapy is an adverse reaction to a therapeutic drug (Brown, pp. 285–300).

72.

C. Combining a prescribed medication with a non-prescribed substance is classified as a poisoning (Brown, p. 335).

73.

A. Combining a prescribed medication with a non-prescribed substance is classified as a poisoning (Brown, p. 335).

74.

D. The patient took the drug as prescribed; therefore, the problems of dizziness and weakness are classified as an adverse reaction, and not poisoning. In addition, the possible cerebrovascular accident was ruled out after the studies revealed the adverse reaction to the Isordil (Brown, p. 335).

75.

A. "A diagnostic statement of . . . intoxication due to a prescription drug such as . . . lithium without any further qualification usually refers to an adverse effect of a correctly administered prescription drug." Figure 29.1 further clarifies that this question deals with an adverse effect of drugs. If the coder will answer each question in the decision tree, it can be determined that this is an adverse effect, although the patient did not tell the clinic doctor that (s)he was on Eskalith; the Eskalith was taken as prescribed, as was the Aldomet (Brown, p. 335).

76.

D. Refer to Skin Graft and Flap, Split Graft in the CPT index and review codes 15100 to 15121. Code 15100 states, "Split graft, . . . arms, legs, . . . 100 sq cm or less. . . ." Also code the excisional preparation of the recipient site by assigning 15000 (CPT, pp. 53, 513).

77.

B. Refer to Jejunostomy in the CPT Index and review code 44015. It states, "Tube or needle catheter jejunostomy for enteral alimentation. . . ." The term alimentation means "the process of nourishing the body . . ." and enteral means ". . . by way of the intestine" (CPT, pp. 144, 458; Taber's, pp. 64, 645).

78.

B. Refer to Aneurysm Repair, Intracranial Artery and review codes 61705 and 61708. Code 61705 states, "Surgery of aneurysm . . . by intracranial electrothrombosis." The term pterional refers to the anatomic "point of suture of frontal, parietal, temporal, and sphenoid bones" and is not considered for coding purposes. The craniotomy is not assigned a code number because of the note located below the heading, Surgery for Aneurysm, which states, "Includes craniotomy when appropriate for procedure" (CPT, pp. 191, 372; Taber's, p. 1595).

79.

C. Refer to Mastectomy, Modified Radical and review code 19240. It states, "Mastectomy, modified radical, including axillary lymph nodes, with or without pectoralis minor muscle, but excluding pectoralis major muscle." A modified radical mastectomy involves removal of the breast, nipple, areola, overlying skin, and axillary lymph nodes. Next, refer to Reconstruction, Breast, Transverse Rectus Abdominis Myocutaneous Flap and review codes 19367 to 19369. Code 19367 includes "Breast reconstruction with transverse rectus abdominis myocutaneous flap (TRAM), single pedicle, including closure of donor site" (CPT, pp. 58–59, 469, 497; Stedman's, p. 925).

80.

B. Rectus abdominis is a type of muscle. The CPT index entry, Flap, refers the coder to Skin Graft and Flap and review codes 15732 to 15738. Code 15738 states, "Muscle . . . flap; lower extremity." Next, Rotation Flap instructs the coder to see Skin, Adjacent Tissue Transfer. Review codes 14000 to 14350. Code 14040 states, "Adjacent tissue transfer or rearrangement, . . . feet; defect 10 sq cm or less." Next, refer to Split Grafts and review codes 15100 to 15121. Assign codes 15100 and 15101 because the graft was 200 square centimeters. Code 15100 states, "Split graft, . . . feet; 100 sq cm or less. . . ." It is necessary to also assign code 15101 to classify "each additional 100 sq cm. . . ." Next, refer to Amputation, Toe and review codes 28810 to 28825. Code 28810 states, "Amputation, metatarsal, with toe, single." Do not assign a code to the debridement because the note located below the heading Free Skin Grafts states, "includes simple debridement . . ." (CPT, pp. 52–54, 98, 368, 431, 512–513, 516; Stedman's, p. 1003).

81.

C. Refer to Cesarean Delivery, Delivery Only and review code 59514 that states, "Cesarean delivery

only." An attempt at vaginal delivery after previous cesarean section, which then results in another cesarean delivery, would be assigned code 59620 (CPT, pp. 182, 394).

82.

B. The term resection means excision. Refer to Brain, Tumor, Excision and review codes 61510, 61518, 61520 to 61521, 61526 to 61530, 61545, and 62164. Code 61518 states, "Craniectomy for excision of brain tumor . . . posterior fossa . . ." (CPT, pp. 188, 388; Stedman's, p. 1345).

83.

A. Refer to Laparoscopy, Biopsy and review codes 47561 and 49321. Code 47561 states, "Laparoscopy, surgical; with guided transhepatic cholangiography with biopsy." The diagnostic laparoscopy is not coded separately because it is included in the code for the surgical laparoscopy. Note the "separate procedure" parenthetical note, which states, "Some of the listed procedures are commonly carried out as an integral part of a total service, and as such do not warrant separate identification" (CPT, pp. 155, 460).

84.

A. Refer to Appendectomy and review codes 44950 to 44960. Code 44950 states, "Appendectomy" (CPT, pp. 147, 375).

85.

C. Refer to Excision, Lesion, Finger and review code 26160 that states, "Excision of lesion . . . (e.g. . . . ganglion), hand or finger" (CPT, pp. 83, 423).

86.

D. Refer to Excision, Lesion, Skin, Malignant and review codes 11600 to 11646. Code 11606 states, "Excision, malignant lesion, trunk, arms . . . lesion diameter over 4.0 cm" (CPT, pp. 49, 424).

87.

D. Refer to Excision, Lesion, Skin, Malignant and review codes 11600 to 11646. Code 11644 states, "Excision, malignant lesion, face. . . lesion diameter 3.1 to 4.0 cm." The wound closure is not coded because the excision code includes simple closure (CPT, pp. 49, 424).

88.

B. Refer to Cast, Long Arm and review code 29065. Assign code 29065 because the fracture was treated (patient transported for definitive care). The cast was applied for "patient comfort during transport." Refer to the notes located below the category, Application of Casts and Strapping. "The listed procedures apply when the cast application is . . . an initial service performed without a restorative treatment . . . to stabilize or protect a fracture . . . and/or to afford comfort to a patient" (CPT, pp. 99, 392).

89.

B. Refer to Sigmoidoscopy, Exploration in the CPT index and review codes 45330 and 45335. Code 45330 states, "Sigmoidoscopy . . ." (CPT, pp. 148, 511).

90.

A. Refer to Excision, Lesion, Skin, Malignant and review codes 11600 to 11646. Code 11643 states, "Excision, malignant lesion, face . . ., lesion diameter 2.1 to 3.0 cm" (CPT, pp. 49, 424).

91.

D. When heart disease or cardiovascular disease is specified as hypertensive, the codes are combined as hypertensive heart disease (Brown, p. 265).

92.

D. "When the diagnostic statement includes both hypertension and renal disease, ICD-9-CM often assumes there is a cause-and-effect relationship. A code from category 403, Hypertensive Renal Disease, is provided in the Alphabetic Index; a causal relationship need not be indicated in the diagnostic statement." Cardiomegaly is not listed as a condition included under category code 403; it also is not stated as hypertensive type and would be coded separately (Brown, p. 265).

93.

C. A late effect requires sequencing of the residual code first, followed by the code for the late effect of the earlier illness (Brown, pp. 43–45).

94.

A. A functioning pacemaker is found in Volume 2 by searching under Status (Buck, Vol. 2, p. 408).

95.

D. Code 193 in Volume 1 of ICD-9-CM instructs the coder to "Use additional code to identify any functional activity." Hypertension is a functional activity and would be coded as secondary hypertension (Buck, Vol. 1, p. 600).

96.

B. This question provides an example of sequencing late effects with the residual first, the late effect of the previous illness second, and the late effect of the external cause last. For the procedure, refer to the ICD-9-CM Index to Procedures' main term, Z-plasty, and subterms, skin (scar) . . ., with excision of lesion, and assign code 86.3 (Brown, pp. 43–45; Buck, Vol. 3, p. 1030).

97.

A. An E code is assigned to classify the external cause of injuries and is never sequenced as the principal diagnosis (Brown, p. 61).

98.

B. A missile fracture is listed as a type of open fracture (Buck, Vol. 1, p. 201).

99.

C. Pathological fractures are classified in Chapter 13 of ICD-9-CM (Diseases of the Musculoskeletal System and Connective Tissue), not Chapter 17 (Injury and Poisoning) (Brown, pp. 196–197, 316).

100.

B. The third-degree burns of the chest and abdomen are classified as multiple sites and are assigned combination code 942.39. Code only the third-degree burns for the left arm, left leg, and abdomen (943.30, 945.20, 945.30). Assign code 948.52 to classify a total body involvement of 50% (fourth digit 5) with 20% third-degree burns (fifth digit 2) (Brown, pp. 330–331).

101.

D. "When a burn is described as infected, two codes are required. The code for the burn is sequenced first, with code 958.3, Post-traumatic wound infection, not elsewhere classified, assigned as an additional code" (Brown, p. 332).

102.

A. The gross hematuria with clots is the result of the presence of the suprapubic bladder tube; this is considered a complication due to presence of an internal device, implant, or graft and is assigned code 996.76. The procedure performed included cystoscopy and evacuation of blood clots; assign codes 57.32 and 57.0. Code 57.93 is not assigned because it includes that "for control of (postoperative) hemorrhage of bladder," which is not included in the procedural statement (Brown, pp. 346–347; Buck, Vol. 3, pp. 1081).

103.

D. Assign multiple codes to classify the multiple sclerosis and paraplegia. Code 340 by itself does not "fully identify the component elements of a complex" diagnosis such as multiple sclerosis. Do not assign a code to the symptom, weakness, because "codes . . . are assigned as secondary codes only when the symptom[s] . . . is not integral to the underlying condition and when its presence makes a difference in the severity of the patient's underlying condition and/or the care given" (Brown, pp. 73–75).

104.

D. Paralytic ileus is a postoperative complication that affects the digestive system and is not classified elsewhere (Brown, p. 343).

105.

A. The peritonitis is an infection that occurred as a complication of a mechanical device, or, in this case, the catheter inserted into the abdomen for ambulatory peritoneal dialysis. Reference ICD-9-CM, Volume 2, main term Complication, and subterms infection and inflammation, due to . . ., catheter . . ., vascular NEC, and assign code 996.62. When verifying code 996.62 in the tabular list, note that the code includes Vascular catheter . . . (dialysis) (Brown, pp. 340–347; Buck, Vol. 1, p. 837; Vol. 2, p. 100).

106.

B. Bowenoid Senile Keratosis is "any condition of the skin characterized by the formation of horny growths or excessive development of the horny growth." Refer to Excision, Lesion, Skin, Benign in the CPT index and review codes 11400 to 11471. Code 11442 states, "Excision, other benign lesion . . . face . . . lesion diameter 1.1 to 2.0 cm" (CPT, pp. 49, 424; Taber's, p. 1046).

107.

D. Refer to Excision, Lesion, Skin, Benign in the CPT index and review codes 11400 to 11471. Assign codes 11441 and 11442 because two lesions were removed, a 1 cm lesion and a 2 × 1 cm lesion. For the 2 × 1 cm lesion, code the excision according to the largest size (CPT, pp. 49, 424).

108.

C. Refer to Biopsy, Bone Marrow in the CPT index and review code 38221. It states, "Bone marrow biopsy, needle or trocar" (CPT, p. 382).

109.

B. Refer to Excision, Lesion, Skin, Malignant in the CPT index and review codes 11600 to 11646. Code 11602 refers to a 2 cm lesion excision (CPT, pp. 49, 424).

110.

A. Refer to Cholecystectomy in the CPT index and review codes 47600 to 47620 and 47562 to 47564. Assign code 47600. Refer to Appendectomy in the CPT index and review codes 44950 to 44960. Do not assign a code for the appendectomy because "Incidental appendectomy during intra-abdominal surgery does not usually warrant a separate identification . . ." (CPT, pp. 147, 153, 375, 396).

111.

D. Refer to Angioplasty, Coronary Artery, Percutaneous Transluminal in the CPT index and review codes 92982 to 92984. Assign code 92982 because it refers to single vessel angioplasty (CPT, pp. 303, 372).

112.

A. Refer to Biopsy, Endometrium in the CPT index and review codes 58100 and 58558. Assign code 58100 because no laparoscopy was performed (CPT, p. 383).

113.

D. Refer to Hysterectomy, Abdominal, Total in the CPT index and review codes 58150 and 58200. Code 58150 states, "Total abdominal hysterectomy . . . with or without removal of tube(s), with or without removal of ovary(s)" (CPT, pp. 178, 446).

114.

B. Although the fracture is stated as open, code it as a closed treatment because it does not state open treatment. Refer to Fracture, Tibia, Closed Treatment in the CPT index and review codes 27530 to 27532, 27538, 27750 to 27752, 27760 to 27762,

27808 to 27810, and 27824 to 27825. Code 27752 states, "Closed treatment of tibial shaft fracture . . . with manipulation, with or without skeletal traction" (CPT, pp. 94, 434).

115.

C. Refer to Fracture, Wrist, with Dislocation, Closed Treatment in the CPT index, review and assign code 25680. In the CPT index, refer to Wound, Repair, Simple and review codes 12001 to 12021. Assign code 12001; it states, "Simple repair of superficial wound of . . . extremities (including hands and feet); 2.5 cm or less" (CPT, pp. 51, 82, 434, 542).

116.

A. Refer to Laparoscopy, Removal, Ovaries in the CPT index and review code 58661. It states, "Laparoscopy, surgical; with . . . (partial or total oophorectomy and/or salpingectomy)" (CPT, pp. 180, 461).

117.

C. Refer to Cesarean Delivery, Delivery Only in the CPT index and review code 59514. It states, "Cesarean delivery only" (CPT, pp. 182, 394)

118.

A. Refer to Bypass Graft, Coronary Artery, Arterial in the CPT index and review codes 33533 to 33536. Assign code 33534 that states, "Coronary artery bypass, using arterial graft(s); two coronary arterial grafts" (CPT, pp. 115, 390).

119.

D. Refer to Laparoscopy, Vaginal Hysterectomy in the CPT index and review code 58550. It states, "Laparoscopy, surgical; with vaginal hysterectomy with or without removal of tube(s), with or without removal of ovary(s) (laparoscopic assisted vaginal hysterectomy)." The bilateral salpingo-oophorectomy is included in code 58550 (CPT, p. 461).

120.

B. Refer to Chemotherapy, Intravenous in the CPT index and review codes 96408 to 96414. Assign

code 96410 that states, "Chemotherapy administration, intravenous; infusion technique, up to one hour." Also assign code 96412 twice to indicate 2 additional hours of chemotherapy administration. Finally, assign code 96545 for "Provision of chemotherapy agent" (CPT, pp. 318–319, 395).

6 Statistics and Data Literacy

objectives

After completion of this chapter, the student will be able to:

- Explain the purpose of collection of vital statistics in health care.

- Compute rates, ratios, proportions, and percentages.

- Compute measures of central tendency and dispersion.

- Explain the basic and advanced health care statistics that are used in the health care field.

- Discuss the methods to display health care data.

- Determine the most appropriate use of the various data presentation techniques.

- Conceptualize the fundamentals of descriptive statistics and data validity and reliability.

DIRECTIONS (Questions 1–60): Each of the questions or incomplete statements below is followed by suggested answers or completions. Select the **best** answer in each case.

1. Which unit of measure suggests services received by one inpatient in one 24-hour period?
   A. an average daily census day
   B. an inpatient service day
   C. the inpatient census
   D. a unit of service day

2. Which meets the requirements of a "low birth weight neonate?"
   A. 5,000 grams or less
   B. 2,500 grams or less
   C. 3,500 grams or less
   D. 2,000 grams or less

3. Which determines whether a fetal death is reportable?
   A. number of weeks of gestation at which the fetus was expelled or extracted
   B. weight of the dead fetus upon expulsion or extraction from the mother
   C. lack of breathing or other evidence of life at the time of expulsion or extraction
   D. the fact that the fetus is preterm at expulsion or extraction from the mother

4. Which is excluded when calculating the net autopsy rate?
   A. inpatient deaths occurring less than 48 hours after admission
   B. infant deaths that occur within the acute care facility
   C. hospital patients whose bodies are unavailable for autopsy
   D. unautopsied medical examiners' cases

5. When compiling a long-term care facility's length of stay statistics, a 24-hour leave of absence is included
   A. each time the L.O.S. statistic is calculated

   B. for inpatient long-term care facility residents only
   C. as determined by long-term care facility policy
   D. if the resident was under a doctor's supervision

6. A hospital sends its ambulance in response to a call. The patient is DOA and is
   A. included in the gross death rate
   B. not included in any inpatient death rates
   C. counted as dead under 48 hours
   D. registered as an outpatient

7. What is the ratio of inpatient service days to inpatient bed count days for a given period of time called?
   A. inpatient census
   B. percent of occupancy
   C. bed turnover rate
   D. average length of stay

8. Discharge days are used in computing the
   A. percent of occupancy
   B. average length of stay
   C. inpatient census
   D. gross autopsy rate

9. Bed turnover rate statistics measure the
   A. number of inpatients present
   B. hospital's utilization
   C. inpatient beds occupied
   D. services received by inpatients

10. The net death rate is the ratio of inpatient deaths during any given period of time to the total number of discharges (and deaths) during that time, and
    A. is a statistic that is not calculated as it does not provide useful information

B. should also include deaths occurring before and after 48 hours of admission

C. is called "gross death rate," also known as "hospital death rate"

D. is an incorrect formula and should exclude "(and deaths)"

11. The major problem with comparing statistics reported by different hospitals because of differences in definitions of various terms used in compiling statistics was reduced when the American Health Information Management Association developed the

A. Uniform Hospital Discharge Data Set

B. Glossary of Health Care Terms

C. Health Care Field Guide

D. L.T.C. Minimum Data Set

12. A neonate whose birth occurs before the end of the last day of the 38th week following the onset of the last menstrual period is termed a

A. immature neonate

B. post-term neonate

C. preterm neonate

D. term neonate

13. The term *census* is defined as the number of inpatients/residents

A. occupying beds in the facility at midnight

B. discharged within a 24-hour period

C. admitted within a 24-hour period

D. present in the facility at any one time

14. The daily analysis of hospital service is based on

A. admissions

B. inpatients and outpatients

C. discharges

D. census

15. A man was injured in an automobile accident and brought to the emergency room of the hospital. He died in the emergency room before treatment could be started. In compiling hospital statistics, this patient would be counted as

A. dead on arrival

B. inpatient death

C. outpatient death

D. institutional death

16. The name of the program that the JCAHO has established for the purpose of data transmission by accredited health care facilities to the accrediting agency is called the

A. Accreditation Manual

B. Conditions of Participation

C. Guide to the Health Care Field

D. Indicator Monitoring System

17. Health care facility statistics about professional work performed are collected and furnished to users for a variety of reasons (e.g., for the purpose of adding nursing staff, closing a nursing unit, offering additional physical therapy services, etc.). It is essential that the facility's administrator, health information professional, and medical staff

A. have a mutual understanding about the definition of terms used, data collected, and accuracy of information

B. compare their health care facility's statistics to those of another facility located in a different state

C. utilize only the health record as the source of data for gathering statistical information at the facility

D. on a daily basis, question the necessity of data collection and report compilation as prepared by the facility

18. In computing long-term care statistics, leaves of absence are excluded for all EXCEPT:

A. inpatient service days calculations

B. patient census calculations

C. bed occupancy calculations

D. length of stay calculations

19. The November 1 inpatient midnight census was 98. On November 2, seven patients were admitted, there was one fetal death as well as one DOA, and nine patients were discharged; one of the discharged patients was admitted at 7:00 A.M. and remained for 8 hours. Calculate the inpatient service days for November 2.

    A. 96
    B. 97
    C. 98
    D. 99

20. The number of available inpatient beds (occupied and vacant) on a given day is called the

    A. inpatient bed count
    B. percentage of occupancy
    C. daily census
    D. inpatient bed count day

21. The daily census includes all of the following EXCEPT:

    A. inpatients/residents present at the census-taking time each day
    B. newborns delivered that day in the acute care facility
    C. patients in an intensive care unit located within the hospital
    D. patients seen in the emergency department of the facility

22. In computing the gross death rate for a hospital, which would be EXCLUDED?

    A. deaths under 48 hours
    B. fetal deaths
    C. coroners' cases
    D. deaths over 48 hours

23. Which statistic would be used to test the validity of data?

    A. range
    B. standard deviation
    C. t-test
    D. variance

24. When developing an in-house computerized discharged inpatient abstracting system, the facility should use the

    A. DHHS
    B. Delphi Technique
    C. MUMPS
    D. UHDDS

25. A baby born in the ambulance on the way to the hospital and admitted is classified as a (an)

    A. pediatric inpatient
    B. newborn inpatient
    C. newborn outpatient
    D. emergency patient

26. Distribution of Patients by Birth Year
    Prior to 1900 2,331
    1901–1925 3,309
    1925–1949 3,118
    1950–1975 4,073
    1976–2000 2,779

    What is the error in the construction of the table above?

    A. too few classes are represented in the table
    B. too many classes are represented in the table
    C. a data item may go into more than one class
    D. a data item may not go into more than one class

27. The complexity of patients treated in a facility, categorized by type and volume, is the

    A. census
    B. case-mix
    C. blended rate
    D. severity of illness

28. A facility's lengths of stay for the month of January include the following: 1, 2, 3, 4, 5, 6,

7, 10, 13, 16, and 30. Determine the range of January's length of stay data.

A. 6

B. 8.8

C. 29

D. 97

29. On August 15, 13 patients were discharged. The LOS for each patient was 17, 3, 4, 25, 8, 7, 13, 10, 5, 11, 9, 21, and 1 day, respectively. The median LOS for these patients was

A. 9.0

B. 11.1

C. 10.3

D. 9.8

30. The lengths of stay for 10 patients discharged in one day were 15, 4, 9, 2, 469, 12, 6, 8, 8, and 11 days. Which measure would best determine the norm for length of service in this unit?

A. arithmetic mean

B. mode

C. median

D. standard deviation

31. Fetal deaths are

A. included in gross and net death rates

B. not included in either gross or net death rates

C. included in the gross death rate, not in the net death rate

D. included in both gross and net death rates when delivery occurs in the hospital

32. Which will best ensure the quality of statistics compiled by a facility?

A. improvement in the quality of health record documentation

B. calculating statistics via computer rather than manually

C. increasing the number of statistical computations required by the facility

D. computing statistics from secondary health records

33. "A period in a person's life during which he is an inpatient in a single hospital without interruption except by possible intervening leaves of absence" is the definition of

A. inpatient admission

B. inpatient hospitalization

C. hospital inpatient

D. nursing facility inpatient

DIRECTIONS: Questions 34–37 refer to the following statistics. (Note: Carry computations to two decimal places and round answers to the nearest tenth). The hospital (410 beds and 60 bassinets) discharged 1,274 adult and child inpatients and 322 newborn infants during September. There were 8,482 patient days of service at the time of discharge for the adult/child patients, and 1,154 patient days of service at discharge for newborn infants. September's census days were 9,173 for adults/children; 1,265 for newborn infants.

---

34. What was the average length of stay, in days, for adults and children?

A. 6.5

B. 6.7

C. 7.0

D. 7.2

35. What was the percent of occupancy of newborn bassinets during September?

A. 21.0%

B. 64.1%

C. 70.3%

D. 91.2%

36. What was the average daily census for adults and children for September?

A. 283

B. 305.8

C. 306

D. 348

37. What was the percent of occupancy of adult and child beds for the month?
    A. 66.7%
    B. 68.8%
    C. 72.2%
    D. 74.6%

DIRECTIONS: Questions 38–39 refer to the following statistics. (Note: Carry computations to two decimal places and round answers to the nearest tenth.) The hospital had 1,244 discharges in January, including 20 deaths. Fourteen of the deaths occurred 48 hours or more after admission; 13 cases were autopsied in the hospital. One death under 48 hours was a medical examiner's case, removed from the hospital for post-mortem exam elsewhere.

---

38. What was the net autopsy rate?
    A. 63.2%
    B. 65.0%
    C. 68.4%
    D. 100%

39. What was the gross death rate?
    A. 1.1%
    B. 1.6%
    C. 11.4%
    D. 16.0%

DIRECTIONS: Questions 40–41 refer to the following statistics. (Note: Carry computations to two decimal places and round answers to the nearest tenth.) In 1997, the hospital's adult inpatient bed capacity was 220 from January 1 to June 30 and 275 from July 1 to December 31. There were 5,996 discharges and 41,972 discharge days from January 1 to June 30 and 6,123 discharges with 42,861 discharge days from July 1 through December 31. From January to June, 37,985 days of service were provided to adult inpatients, and from July to December, 48,542 adult inpatient days of service were rendered.

---

40. What was the percent of occupancy of adult beds for the year?
    A. 91.8%

B. 93.0%
C. 95.2%
D. 95.7%

41. Calculate the total length of stay for all adult inpatients in 1997.
    A. 12,119
    B. 75,970
    C. 84,833
    D. 86,527

DIRECTIONS: Questions 42–43 refer to the following statistics. (Note: Carry computations to two decimal places and round answers to the nearest tenth.) The hospital discharged 13,642 patients during 1997. There were 225 deaths, with 100 of them occurring under 48 hours. Total autopsies performed for the year were 75. Ten of the 225 deaths were medical examiners' cases that could not be autopsied at the hospital. There were also 63 fetal deaths, and 11 autopsies were performed on the fetal deaths.

---

42. What was the gross death rate for the year?
    A. 0.9%
    B. 1.6%
    C. 17.4%
    D. 4.4%

43. What was the hospital autopsy rate for the year?
    A. 40%
    B. 33.3%
    C. 34.9%
    D. 27%

44. The minimum common core of data required on hospital Medicare/Medicaid patients is the
    A. Uniform Hospital Discharge Data Set
    B. Uniform Patient Discharge Data Set
    C. Medicare/Medicaid Patient Discharge Data Set
    D. Medicare/Medicaid Hospital Data Set

45. Registration of births, deaths, and fetal deaths is governed by
    A. federal laws
    B. state civil laws
    C. county regulations
    D. United States Public Health Service

46. Copies of vital certificates are ultimately forwarded to the
    A. National Center for Disease Control
    B. World Health Organization
    C. Federal Office of Vital Statistics
    D. National Center for Health Statistics

47. A hospital intensive care unit (ICU) wishes to compute the ratio of its patients that were treated with mechanical ventilators during the past month. The correct formula is

    A. $\dfrac{\text{No. of ICU patients on ventilators during the period}}{\text{No. of all hospital patients on ventilators during the period} \times 100}$

    B. $\dfrac{\text{No. of all patients in the ICU during the period}}{\text{No. of patients on ventilators during the period} \times 100}$

    C. $\dfrac{\text{No. of ICU patients on ventilators during the period}}{\text{No. of all patients in the ICU during the period} \times 100}$

    D. $\dfrac{\text{No. of ICU patients on ventilators during the period}}{\text{No. of ICU patients not on ventilators during the period} \times 100}$

48. The AHA publishes an annual survey of hospitals in order to produce the
    A. Accreditation Manual for Hospitals
    B. Hospital Survey Profile
    C. Guide to the Health Care Field
    D. Directory of Residency Training Programs

49. When personnel visit a hospital nursing station to collect data from inpatient health records, this is called
    A. retrospective review
    B. concurrent review
    C. discharge analysis
    D. service analysis

50. In any computerized data collection system
    A. there is actually too much data collected to provide accurate reporting mechanisms
    B. computerized information processing requires quality control checks to be performed
    C. there is never enough data collected to provide optimal reliability in computations
    D. accuracy of data collected is consistent with the number of people collecting data

51. Which graphical presentation type always depicts percentages?
    A. bar graph
    B. pie graph
    C. histogram
    D. line graph

52. The facility's statistics reveal a recent change in the average length of stay for inpatients. Last year, lengths of stay averaged 4.1 days. This year, the average length of stay is 4.3 days. The standard deviation last year was 16 and this year it is 14. What is the interpretation of this data?
    A. each discharged patient's length of stay values are closer to the average LOS value of 4.3 this year as compared to last year's data
    B. the facility's inpatient average length of stay variance is 0.2 days, which indicates that the average length of stay is increasing
    C. more inpatients had an average length of stay of 4.1 days last year as compared with this year's average length of stay of 4.3 days
    D. Average lengths of stay are much greater this year for inpatients as compared with the same statistical data last year

53. Nursing personnel have recently been required to input TPR (temperature, pulse, and respiration) data into the facility's computerized health record system. To get the nursing staff to realize the value of this computerized input of data, you have convinced the computer center to create an onscreen graphical display of this information. Because TPR information is input continuously on each patient, which would be the best choice for displaying the information?
    A. pie chart
    B. line graph
    C. rate/ratio
    D. variance

54. Upon analysis of the increased incidence of heart disease cases in a particular region of the country, the epidemiologist prepared a report including recommendations as to the need for additional preventive measures with regard to the disease. The incidence of heart disease cases is the number of
    A. heart disease cases receiving treatment within the population
    B. newly diagnosed heart disease cases last year within the population
    C. known heart disease cases at the present time within the population
    D. current heart disease cases who need medical and social care to cope

55. In general, graphs
    A. have less appeal than tables of numerical listings
    B. are extremely complex in presentation
    C. should contain as much information as possible
    D. help the reader understand information more quickly

56. A study that can be repeated with the same results is considered to be
    A. valid
    B. sound
    C. reliable
    D. cogent

57. When gathering data about pediatric patients age 13 or younger, it would be best to
    A. classify them as pediatric patients only if cared for by an organized medical staff unit of pediatrics
    B. allow each medical staff service (e.g., general practice, internal medicine, etc.) to determine the age to be used
    C. use the broadest grouping of ages whenever possible when gathering information on this patient population
    D. comply with federal regulations dictating that pediatric patient data be gathered separately from adult data

58. The hospital's governing board is to determine whether the facility should expand its inpatient bed capacity. Which statistical information would best assist the governing board in its decision making?
    A. hospital discharge days
    B. daily inpatient census
    C. average length of stay
    D. percent of occupancy

59. One way to determine the validity of data collected in an empirical study would be to use a statistical measure such as a (an)
    A. mean
    B. t-test
    C. table
    D. variance

60. It would be appropriate to use a bar graph to present data if
    A. the categories of data displayed are not continuous
    B. numerical data are first converted to percentages before displaying it
    C. the data presented must be adjacent to each other on the graph
    D. data are represented by dots placed over midpoints on the display

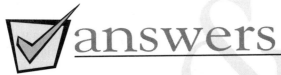
1.

B. An inpatient service day is also known as a resident service day (Youmans, p. 13).

2.

D. A low birth weight neonate is a live born infant with a birth weight of less than, but not equal to, 2,500 grams. This rules out **B.** as the answer because the infant cannot weigh 2,500 grams (Brown, p. 239).

3.

C. A fetal death occurs before the complete expulsion or extraction from the mother of a product of conception, fetus, and placenta. The duration of the pregnancy is not a consideration in determining fetal death. Lack of respirations or other evidence of life indicates death after extraction or expulsion of the fetus (Brown, p. 223).

4.

D. The net autopsy rate formula is:

$$\frac{\text{Total inpatient autopsies in a given period}}{\text{Total inpatient deaths—unautopsied}} \times 100$$
medical examiners' cases

This rate includes the number of autopsies performed only on inpatients by the hospital's pathology department. Newborn (infant) autopsies and deaths are included in autopsy rates. All deaths of inpatients are included. Answer **C.** implies that hospital patients other than inpatients should be considered (e.g., emergency department patients); however, these patients are included in the hospital or adjusted autopsy rate, which includes all autopsies, inpatient or otherwise, that have been performed by the hospital's pathology department (Youmans, p. 66).

5.

C. The long-term care facility determines the policy as to whether leaves of absence are counted as a continuous stay or separately calculated when determining length of stay statistics (Youmans, p. 87).

6.

B. This patient would be considered dead on arrival (DOA), and should not be considered as a patient of the hospital (either inpatient or outpatient). The hospital death rates concern only inpatients (Youmans, p. 61).

7.

B. The formula for percent of occupancy (also called the inpatient bed occupancy ratio) is:

$$\frac{\text{Total inpatient service days for a period}}{\text{Total inpatient bed count days in the period} \times 100}$$

(Youmans, pp. 29–30).

8.

B. Average length of stay is the correct answer. Discharge days are compiled on the patient after he or she has been discharged from the hospital. LOS is a synonymous term for discharge days (Youmans, p. 38).

9.

B. The bed turnover rate indicates the impact that changes in percent of occupancy rates and length of

101

stay have on the facility in terms of bed utilization (Youmans, pp. 32–33).

10.

C. The gross death rate (or hospital death rate) uses the formula described in the question:

$$\frac{\text{Number of deaths of inpatients in a given period}}{\text{Number of discharges including deaths in that period}} \times 100$$

The net death rate is not routinely calculated today because the distinction between deaths over and under 48 hours of admission is not really useful (Abdelhak, pp. 60–61, Youmans, p. 60).

11.

B. To improve uniformity in statistical definitions, the American Health Information Management Association most recently developed the 2000 edition of the Glossary of Healthcare Terms (Youmans, p. 139).

12.

C. A low birth weight neonate is any neonate whose weight at birth is less than 2,500 gm. A term neonate's birth occurs from the first day of the 39th week through the last day of the 42nd week. A post-term neonate's birth occurs from the first day of the 43rd week (Brown, pp. 240–241).

13.

D. The question refers to the Glossary of Healthcare Terms (American Health Information Management Association, 2000) definition of the general term *census* (Youmans, pp. 10, 144).

14.

C. A daily analysis of hospital service is based on the patients discharged that day. The discharge analysis should describe the activities of the medical staff units (services) in the hospital. Many facilities have incorporated this data collection in their automated abstracting system (Abdelhak, pp. 319–320; Youmans, pp. 38–39).

15.

C. A patient who dies in the emergency room is considered an inpatient death only when the patient has been admitted to the hospital as an inpatient; that is, the patient is being held in the emergency room until a bed in the area of the hospital where patients stay overnight is ready. Even if treatment had begun but the patient had not been admitted, the patient would have been considered an outpatient or emergency room death (Youmans, pp. 60–61).

16.

D. The Accreditation Manual is produced by the Joint Commission for facility reference in preparation for the accreditation process. Conditions of Participation are produced by HCFA for use in implementing the Medicare and Medicaid programs. The Guide to the Health Care Field is a publication prepared by the American Hospital Association and contains data on organization structure, facilities and services, beds and utilization by inpatient services, financial status, personnel, and medical staff (Abdelhak, p. 376).

17.

A. It is essential that data collected be relevant, reliable, and periodically reviewed, and that the health record be used in data compilation. Statistics have added meaning when they are compared to a previous year's statistics within a health care facility or that the same year's statistics be compared with those of a different health care facility (Abdelhak, pp. 106–107, 153–154, 393–394; Johns, pp. 36, 161).

18.

D. Since leaves of absence are usually considered part of one continuous stay, the days involved are usually included in length of stay computations (Youmans, pp. 38, 42).

19.

B. In this situation, 98 patients + 7 admitted patients = 105. The fetal death and the DOA are not admitted patients and are not counted in the census. Thus,

105 patients − 9 discharges = 96 patients. Each of the 96 patients received one day of service = 96 inpatient service days. The 96 inpatient service days + 1 for the patient who was admitted and discharged on November 2 = 97 inpatient service days for November 2 (Youmans, pp. 13–14).

20.

A. An inpatient bed count day is a unit of measure indicating that one bed is set up and ready for occupancy for one day. The inpatient bed count, however, denotes the total number of beds set up and ready for occupancy on a given day and is the correct answer here (Youmans, p. 29).

21.

D. Emergency Department patients are ambulatory patients (Abdelhak, pp. 21, 30).

22.

B. Fetal deaths are not included in death rates (except for a special fetal death rate that a hospital might wish to compute). The gross death rate (or hospital death rate) refers to all inpatient deaths, and includes newborn deaths but not fetal deaths. The net or institutional death rate excludes deaths under 48 hours. Exclusion of coroners' cases occurs only in autopsy rates, not in death rates (Youmans, p. 60).

23.

C. The t-test is a commonly used statistic to test validity. The t-test analyzes the statistical significance between the means of two groups. Range, variance, and standard deviation are measures of variation, not validity (Abdelhak, pp. 328, 331–332; Johns, pp. 426–428).

24.

D. DHHS is the abbreviation for the Department of Health and Human Services, which developed the Uniform Hospital Discharge Data Set (UHDDS). The Delphi Technique is a method of brainstorming used in problem solving. MUMPS (Massachusetts General Hospital Utility Multi-Programming System) is a high-level computer language designed for use with medical application software (Abdelhak, pp. 79, 173; Johns, p. 109).

25.

A. Newborn inpatients must be born in the hospital. Babies born at home or on the way to the hospital are usually placed on the pediatric service (if there is no pediatric service, they are placed on the medical service) (Abdelhak, pp. 90, 96).

26.

C. Birth year data is subdivided into five classes in this example. The number of classes in a frequency distribution table should be determined by the needs of the users of the data. The question of how many should be represented in the example is not answerable because we do not know why these data are being displayed. Note the overlap between classes two and three; it would be difficult to determine where data relevant to date of birth in 1925 would be recorded (Abdelhak, pp. 322–323).

27.

B. The categorization (type and volume) of patients treated in the hospital representing the complexity of its case load is called the case-mix (Abdelhak, p. 634; Johns, p. 371).

28.

C. The range is determined by subtracting the smallest value in a set of numbers from the largest. In this question, 6 represents the median, 8.8 is the mean, and 97 is the total of all of the lengths of stay. (Abdelhak, p. 328; Johns, p. 426).

29.

A. To find the median, the data must be arranged in numerical order: 1, 3, 4, 5, 7, 8, 9, 10, 11, 13, 17, 21, 25. The median is the middle data element in this array; or, if there is an even number of data elements, the average of the two data elements nearest the middle. Since there are 13 data elements in this array (i.e., 13 patients were discharged), we need to find the seventh data element, or 9.0 in this example (Abdelhak, p. 327; Johns, pp. 424–425).

30.

C. The median is the most appropriate measure because the longest length of stay of 469 distorts the arithmetic mean. The mode, or most commonly occurring data element, cannot be computed because none of the data elements has the same value as another. The standard deviation is a measure of variability of the data around the mean, and although it might provide some useful information about the norm for the length of stay on this unit, it would have to be used in combination with the mean (Abdelhak, pp. 326–328; Johns, pp. 422–428).

31.

B. A fetal death is not considered an inpatient death because the fetus did not live at any time after birth. Only inpatients (usually including newborns) are included in gross and net death rates (Youmans, pp. 48–49).

32.

A. This illustrates the idea of choosing the "best answer." Quality in statistical compilation implies that accurate data are being used to compute the statistics. Statistics are only as good as their sources. Because the patient record is the primary data source for health facility statistics, improvements in quality documentation lead to better-quality statistics. Answer B is not necessarily true because input into the computer can be incorrect; a careful statistician can be as accurate as a computer and provide the same quality. Considerable time can be saved by using a computer, however. Answer C can have the opposite effect because increasing the number of statistics kept can reduce quality due to less time and other resources being devoted to each statistical compilation. Because secondary health records are derived from the primary patient record, answer A is better than D (Abdelhak, p. 308).

33.

B. Inpatient admission is when a patient is provided with room, board, and continuous nursing service

in an area of the hospital where patients generally stay at least overnight. Hospital patient or nursing facility patient would refer to the individual (the patient), not the period of time (Abdelhak pp. 540–541).

34.

B. The formula for average length of stay is (Youmans, p. 40):

$$\frac{\text{Total length of stay (discharge days)}}{\text{Total discharges}}$$

In this case (adults and children only; average length of stay for newborns is reported separately):

$$\frac{8,482}{1,274} = 6.66 = 6.7 \text{ days}$$

35.

C. The formula for percent of occupancy is:

$$\frac{\text{Total inpatient service days (or census days) for a period} \times 100}{\text{Total inpatient bed count days} \times \text{number of days in the period}}$$

In this problem (newborn bassinets only, 30 days in September

$$\frac{1,265 \times 100 =}{60 \times 30} \quad \frac{1,265 \times 100}{1,800} = 70.27 = 70.3\%$$

It is important to understand that patient days of service recorded at the time of discharge is equivalent to discharge days or length of stay and is not used in calculating percent of occupancy. Instead, use the figure for census days (another term for inpatient service days). Other names for inpatient service day are inpatient day and bed occupancy day (Youmans, pp. 29–30).

36.

C. The formula is:

$$\frac{\text{Total inpatient service days for a period}}{\text{Total number of days in the period}}$$

In this problem (adults and children only, 30 days in September):

$$\frac{9,173}{30} = 305.77 = 306$$

Again, the figure for census days or inpatient service days must be used: 9,173. Because we are calculating an answer involving persons, we must round off to a whole number, despite instructions to round to the nearest tenth. This is a good example of finding the best answer to a question (Youmans, pp. 16–18).

37.

D. The formula is (Youmans, pp. 16–18):

$$\frac{\text{Total inpatient service days for a period} \times 100}{\text{Total inpatient bed count days} \times \text{number of days in the period}}$$

In this problem (using census days):

$$\frac{9{,}173 \times 100}{410 \times 30} = \frac{9{,}173 \times 100}{12{,}300} = 74.58 = 74.6\%$$

38.

C. The formula for net autopsy rate is:

$$\frac{\text{Total inpatient autopsies for a given period} \times 100}{\begin{array}{c}\text{Total inpatient deaths} - \text{unautopsied coroners'} \\ \text{or medical examiners' cases}\end{array}}$$

In this case: $\dfrac{13 \times 100}{20 - 1} = \dfrac{13 \times 100}{19} = 68.42 = 68.4\%$

The fact that death in the medical examiner's case occurred under 48 hours after admission is irrelevant. The net autopsy rate differs from the hospital or adjusted autopsy rate in only one way. In the hospital autopsy, two situations will cause an increase in the denominator: (1) medical examiners' cases for which the hospital pathologist performs the autopsy and (2) autopsies performed in the hospital on other hospital patients who died elsewhere (e.g., ambulatory care patients, hospital home care patients, and former hospital patients) (Youmans, p. 66).

39.

B. The gross (hospital) death rate formula is (Youmans, p. 60):

$$\frac{\text{Number of deaths of inpatients in a period} \times 100}{\text{Number of discharges (including deaths) in the same period}}$$

In this case: $\dfrac{20 \times 100}{1{,}244} = 1.61\% = 1.6\%$

40.

D. The formula for percent of occupancy is (Youmans, p. 30):

$$\frac{\text{Total inpatient service days for a period} \times 100}{\text{Total inpatient bed count} \times \text{number of days in the period}}$$

In this question, we must consider the fact that the hospital bed count changed halfway through the year. The number of days from January 1 to June 30 in a non-leap year is $31 + 28 + 31 + 30 + 31 + 30 = 181$. From July 1 to December 31, it is $31 + 31 + 30 + 31 + 30 + 31 = 184$. The total is 365. From January 1 to June 30, there were 220 beds and 37,985 days of service (or inpatient service days) during 181 days. From July 1 to December 31, there were 275 beds and 48,542 days of service during 184 days. Therefore:

$$\frac{37{,}985 + 48{,}542 \text{ (total inpatient service days)} \times 100}{(220 \text{ beds} \times 181 \text{ days}) + (275 \text{ beds} \times 184 \text{ days})} = 95.69 = 95.7\%$$

41.

C. Total length of stay (or discharge days) is calculated by totaling all inpatient discharge days for a period of time. You would not use inpatient days of service (or census days) for this calculation (answer D) nor total discharges (answer B). Answer A represents the average daily census (237) (Youmans, p. 38).

42.

B. The gross death rate formula is (Youmans, p. 60):

$$\frac{\text{Total inpatient deaths (including newborns)} \times 100}{\text{Total number of discharges (including deaths and newborns)}}$$

In this case: $\dfrac{225 \times 100}{13{,}642} = 1.64 = 1.6\%$

Answer A represents the net death rate (excluding deaths under 48 hours), which is a statistic not used as an indicator of hospital care because distinguishing between gross and net death rates is not useful. Answer C calculates the percentage of medical examiners' cases not autopsied at the hospital and would use the following formula:

$$\frac{\text{Total number of medical examiners' cases} \times 100}{\text{Total inpatient deaths}}$$

43.

C. The formula for hospital (adjusted) autopsy rate is:

$$\frac{\text{Total hospital autopsies} \times 100}{\begin{array}{c}\text{Number of deaths of hospital patients whose} \\ \text{bodies are available for hospital autopsy}\end{array}}$$

In this case, we have to exclude fetal deaths because they are counted separately. We also have to exclude the 10 cases released to the medical examiner from the denominator, because these bodies were not available for hospital autopsy:

$$\frac{75 \times 100}{225 - 10} = 34.88 = 34.9\%$$

(225 inpatient deaths; 10 medical examiner's cases)

Often statistical problems include more information than is needed to solve the problem (as in this case, which included information about fetal deaths and autopsies). It is necessary to determine carefully which figures are needed in the formula (Youmans, pp. 68–69).

44.

A. The UHDDS was revised for discharges in 1986. It includes 14 data items, which are listed in the references (Abdelhak, pp. 113–114; Johns, pp. 109–112).

45.

B. State civil laws govern the registration of births and deaths, as well as the reporting of fetal deaths (Abdelhak, pp. 436–437).

46.

D. The National Center for Health Statistics, part of the Public Health Service of the United States Department of Health and Human Services, receives copies of the original certificates that are sent to the state registrar. The Center compiles statistical reports for the nation as a whole and for each state. Only certain information compiled from the certificates is sent to the World Health Organization, not copies of the certificates themselves. Answer C is a fabrication (Abdelhak, pp. 308–309; Johns, p. 458–466).

47.

C. The formula for computing any ratio is the:

$$\frac{\text{Number of times something did happen} \times 100}{\text{Number of times it could have happened}}$$

Remembering this formula will assist the student in recalling the various established statistical rates, as well as one-time examples such as this one. In this example, theoretically, all the intensive care unit patients could have been treated with mechanical ventilators, so the denominator must include all patients treated in the intensive care unit during the period (Abdelhak, p. 309; Johns, p. 419).

48.

C. The Accreditation Manual for Hospitals (answer A) is the manual of hospital accreditation standards published by the Joint Commission. The Hospital Survey Profile (answer B) is the name of the questionnaire used by the Joint Commission in its accreditation process. The Directory of Residency Training Programs (answer D) is published by the AMA (AHA, p. 1).

49.

B. A concurrent review system involves personnel visiting the nursing floor to collect data from the records while the patient is still an inpatient. Retrospective review involves collecting data upon discharge of the patient from the facility. Discharge analysis involves the review of records after the discharge of the patient from the facility. (It could be completed in the health information management department or on the nursing unit just after discharge of the patient.) Hospital service analysis is used to describe professional activities of the medical staff and/or specialty clinical educational (residencies) programs of the hospital (Abdelhak, p. 44; Johns, p. 771).

50.

B. The health information management department must accept the responsibility to establish quality controls to determine that the computerized input of patient information is accurate and reliable. Answers A and C are incorrect because it is possible to manage a data collection system that produces optimal data to provide for the needs of those using the data. Answer D implies a relationship between the quality (i.e., accuracy, timeliness, type, and amount) of data collected and the number of personnel involved in the data collection process; this may or may not apply depending upon the personnel and their management (Abdelhak, p. 89; Johns, p. 23).

51.

B. Bar graphs represent noncontinuous categories of data; histograms present frequency distributions; line graphs are also known as frequency polygons and display frequency distributions; the pie graph is a display that divides a circle into pie-shaped wedges that represent distribution percentages (Abdelhak, p. 323; Johns, p. 436).

52.

A. Standard deviation data are the key to this answer. When a standard deviation is small, data collected is close in value to the mean (average). In this case, the standard deviation from one year to the next decreased; the current year's patients' lengths of stay were closer to the average length of stay than last year's patients (Abdelhak, pp. 328–329; Johns, pp. 428–429).

53.

B. The line graph allows for midpoints of classes of data to be connected in a line and it would also be possible to read a value (such as a patient's temperature, pulse, or respiration) along the line. A pie chart could be used to represent one set of data (e.g., temperature, pulse, or respiration); the histogram would allow for all data to be pictorially displayed. Rate or ratio and variance represent measures of variation statistics and are not graphic displays (Abdelhak, p. 397; Johns, pp. 437–438).

54.

B. Answer C represents the prevalence of the disease; answers A and D were fabricated. This is an example of incidence rate, which is the rate of new cases for a given population (Abdelhak, p. 359).

55.

D. Graphs facilitate the understanding of data displays. According to Koch, a graph "should not attempt to present so much information that it becomes confusing to the user and is difficult for the user to comprehend" (Abdelhak, p. 323; Koch, p. 164).

56.

C. The terms *valid, cogent,* and *sound* are synonyms. Thus, the scientific method requires a study to be repeatable for reliability purposes (Abdelhak, pp. 350–351).

57.

A. There is no U.S. standard dividing line between children and adults. Most facilities consider patients who are 13 years of age or younger to be children; however, many facilities use age 14 as the cutoff. It is helpful if the actual age of a child is recorded upon admission, but this is not something that can be established by law in a facility. It would be best to consider children pediatric patients if treated by an organized medical staff department (unit) consisting of pediatricians (Abdelhak, p. 28).

58.

D. The percent of occupancy (or inpatient bed occupancy rate) indicates the proportion of inpatient beds occupied, expressed as a percentage. For example, if the percent of occupancy for the hospital is high (above 90%), the facility may want to seriously consider expanding bed size. The other statistics mentioned as responses certainly would provide information to the governing board about utilization of the inpatient services; however, the percent of occupancy will provide the best measure as to whether bed expansion is a viable option. Bed turnover rate would be an additional statistic that the board would want to review (although this was not provided as a choice in response to the question) (Youmans, pp. 29–35).

59.

B. The t-test (or t-score) is a statistical measure used to test validity of data collected (e.g., mean scores of two groups of data); other measures include the z-score, Mann–Whitney U, Runs test, etc. Mean is a measure of central tendency; you would perform the t-test on two sets of means to establish the validity of the data. Variance is a measure of variation; once you have determined the mean of two or more groups of data, you could determine the variance of that data. Variance does not, however, test the validity of the empirical data gathered. A table is a presentation form of the data and it, too, does not test for validity (Abdelhak, pp. 331–332; Johns, pp. 422–428).

60.

A. Bar graphs (or bar charts) are used to display categories of data that are not continuous. Percentages are calculated first when creating a pie graph. A histogram displays data in a contiguous (adjacent) manner. A frequency polygon is a graphic display device that utilizes dots placed over midpoints; the dots are then connected by straight lines (Abdelhak, pp. 323–325; Johns, pp. 434–440).

7 Legal and Ethical Issues

objectives

After completion of this chapter, this student will be able to:

➤ Describe the legal court system.

➤ Explain the legislative process including the parties involved, officers of the court, documents related to a lawsuit, and legal proceedings.

➤ Explain the HIPAA Security Program and its provisions established to protect health information.

➤ Define the legal vocabulary applicable to the health care field.

➤ Discuss the importance of privacy and confidentiality and the legal implications.

➤ Explain retention guidelines applicable to the health care field.

➤ Describe the ethical issues related to patient rights/advocacy and advance directives.

➤ Explain legal aspects and requirements of consents of specific procedures.

➤ Describe authorized and nonauthorized disclosures of patient information including components and circumstances of releasing confidential information.

DIRECTIONS (Questions 1–62): Each of the questions or incomplete statements below is followed by suggested answers or completions. Select the **best** answer in each case.

1. The health record of a hospital patient is the property of the
   A. patient
   B. attending physician
   C. health information management
   D. hospital

2. Microfilmed records may be submitted as primary evidence.
   A. always
   B. only if the original health record has been destroyed
   C. only if the court has the facilities to reproduce the microfilm in hard copy
   D. never

3. When the patient sues the physician, privileged communication is
   A. extended
   B. continued
   C. voided
   D. promoted

4. If a hospital is sued by a patient, the patient's health record may be released to the hospital attorney
   A. only upon receipt of a subpoena duces tecum
   B. only upon receipt of the patient's authorization
   C. only upon receipt of a written authorization from the hospital administrator
   D. without authorization or subpoena duces tecum

5. All of the following might be a problem associated with an authorization to release information EXCEPT:
   A. authorizations to release "any and all" information

   B. authorizations signed retrospectively
   C. authorizations signed prospectively
   D. release of information by the recipient

6. A health information practitioner as a witness is qualified to answer all of the following questions EXCEPT:
   A. who was responsible for compiling each part of the record
   B. the advisability of the treatment provided the patient
   C. whether the record was kept as part of the hospital's regular order of business
   D. what the components of the record are

7. All of the following might be construed as tampering with an entry in the health record EXCEPT:
   A. writing over the entry
   B. erasing the entry
   C. adding marginal notes to the entry
   D. writing over a spelling error in the entry

8. Without the patient's authorization, employers are entitled to
   A. no information except dates of admission and discharge
   B. no information at all from their employees' records
   C. any and all information, provided they will be paying for hospital treatment
   D. no information except identifying information and the prognosis

9. As director of the health information management department, you receive a subpoena duces tecum for the minutes of the hospital's Surgical Review Committee. In the absence of a hospital policy to guide you, you should
   A. honor the subpoena

B. inform the hospital attorney before honoring the subpoena

C. inform the subpoena server that the subpoena must be served on the chairman of the tissue committee

D. inform the Chief of Staff

10. Of the following answers, which one contains a requestor who is NOT required to submit the patient's written authorization or obtain a court order before medical information is released from the patient's health record? (The patient was treated for a myocardial infarction.)

A. Internal Revenue Service, Veterans Administration, county welfare department, attorneys, the police

B. the hospital's Quality Management Committee, commercial health insurance companies, the patient's employer, a life insurance company to which the patient has applied for life insurance

C. the Federal Bureau of Investigation, county sheriff's office, office of the district attorney

D. the local office of the Public Health Department, the local medical society, the patient's spouse, a physician who last treated the patient 3 years ago

11. A document that requires a person to appear at the designated place at the designated time is termed a (an)

A. subpoena

B. subpoena duces tecum

C. primary evidence

D. attorney's subpoena

12. An attorney, with proper authorization from a patient, obtains a copy of the patient's health record. The attorney then releases a copy of the record to a second attorney. This practice is appropriate

A. always

B. never

C. only if the second attorney is representing the patient's physician in a malpractice case

D. if the second attorney has the patient's authorization

13. A written authorization for release of information from the health record of a psychiatric patient might be signed by the patient's

A. attending physician

B. attorney

C. legal representative

D. next of kin

14. The doctrine of res ipsa loquitur can be illustrated in which of the following cases?

A. a surgeon nicking a ureter during tubal ligation

B. a surgeon leaving a surgical instrument in the body unintentionally

C. a surgeon performing an appendectomy on a patient found after surgery to have a normal appendix

D. a nurse neglecting to give postoperative pain medication as ordered

15. The theory of respondeat superior would apply in which of the following situations?

A. when a hospital medical technologist is negligent, the attending physician can be held liable

B. when the attending physician is negligent, the hospital can be held liable

C. when a hospital nurse is negligent, the director of nursing services (or equivalent) can be held liable

D. when a hospital pharmacist is negligent, the hospital can be held liable

16. In most states, the final court of appeals is called the

A. Supreme Court or Court of Appeals

B. District Appeals Court

C. Justice's Court

D. Circuit Court

17. Upon receipt of a subpoena duces tecum, which of the following should be removed from the health record?
    A. correspondence
    B. consent forms
    C. nurses' notes
    D. graphic reports

18. The physician has
    A. the right to restrict release of information from the health record
    B. the right to remove health records from the hospital
    C. no legal right to the health record
    D. the right to restrict the use of his or her records in quality management activity

19. An incident report should be
    A. destroyed within a week of the incident
    B. kept with the health record
    C. kept separate from the health record
    D. kept in the health record but removed if the record is subpoenaed

20. A person against whom an action is brought in a lawsuit is the
    A. appellee
    B. plaintiff
    C. bailiff
    D. defendant

21. A patient who is 17 years old, married, and living apart from his parents should have an authorization for release of information from his health record signed by
    A. himself
    B. either of his parents
    C. his wife
    D. either himself or his wife

22. Placing health records on computer results in increasing the problems related to
    A. maintaining a timely record

B. providing a physical record that can be used in court
C. the number of persons having access to confidential information
D. placing the record on microfilm

23. What a reasonably prudent person would have done under similar circumstances is termed the
    A. duty of the provider
    B. standard of care
    C. patient–physician privilege
    D. common law

24. Refusing to honor a subpoena can result in
    A. being considered in contempt of court
    B. judicial fines being imposed
    C. arrest
    D. another subpoena being issued

25. In the absence of specific regulations, a guideline for the retention of records established jointly by the American Medical Association and the American Health Information Management Association is to keep records for how many years beyond the most recent episode of care?
    A. 15
    B. 10
    C. 7
    D. 25

26. The patient whose life is threatened and who is comatose is assumed to give what kind of consent for life-sustaining treatment?
    A. informed
    B. express
    C. direct
    D. implied

27. The responsibility for securing informed consent to operate rests primarily with the
    A. admitting office

B. surgeon

C. operating room supervisory nurse

D. unit nurse

28. The touching of an individual in a way that is unsettling, provoking, or physically injurious without that individual's consent is called

A. assault

B. willful bodily harm

C. battery

D. malpractice

29. Health records might be held to be inadmissible if the court ruled that they were

A. hearsay evidence

B. primary evidence

C. circumstantial evidence

D. business records

30. The document that gives the defendant or plaintiff a detailed statement of the plaintiff's claim or the defense of the defendant is called the

A. motion

B. examination before trial

C. bill of particulars

D. summons

31. A court of original jurisdiction is one in which

A. cases are brought before being referred to the state level

B. cases and special proceedings are tried

C. cases brought from appellate courts are heard

D. only federal cases are heard

32. The information in the health record is owned by the

A. patient

B. attending physician

C. health information management

D. hospital

33. An attorney, with proper authorization from a patient, obtains a copy of the patient's health record. The attorney then releases a copy of the record to a second attorney. This practice is called

A. rerelease

B. redisclosure

C. retrospective release

D. secondary release

34. A subpoena issued by an attorney

A. can be ignored at the discretion of the hospital attorney

B. must be obeyed

C. must be countersigned by a judge

D. must be countersigned by the clerk of the court or a judge

35. The party who commences a lawsuit is the

A. defendant

B. appellant

C. contestee

D. plaintiff

36. The legal theories that may be used to support a suit for damages for the unauthorized disclosure of information include all of the following EXCEPT:

A. defamation

B. breach of confidentiality

C. invasion of privacy

D. invalidation of consent

37. If a patient has a primary diagnosis of alcoholism, which of the following information items may be released without his or her consent?

A. admission and discharge dates only

B. name only

C. name, address, age, sex, and attending physician only

D. no information, including the fact that he or she was treated at the facility

38. When preparing a health record in response to a subpoena duces tecum, all of the following should be done EXCEPT:
    A. each page should be numbered
    B. each page should be checked to make sure that it contains the patient's name and health record number
    C. the record should be read to see if there is a possibility of a malpractice suit
    D. the attending physician should be notified

39. A written patient authorization should contain all of the following EXCEPT:
    A. the signature of the person requesting the information
    B. the signature of the patient or authorized representative allowing release of information
    C. the purpose of or need for the information
    D. the name of the person or institution that is to receive the information

40. Consent for the release of information about a minor is generally required of the
    A. patient
    B. physician
    C. parent
    D. parent or legal guardian

41. The physician–patient privilege belongs to
    A. the patient
    B. the physician
    C. both the patient and the physician
    D. either the patient or the physician, depending on the circumstances

42. Secondary patient records include all of the following EXCEPT:
    A. indexes
    B. computerized patient registration system
    C. registers
    D. financial data

43. A subpoena should be refused in all of the following cases EXCEPT:
    A. when the signature of the patient is not present on the subpoena
    B. when the date, time, and place of appearance are not stated on the subpoena
    C. when the signature of the official empowered to issue the subpoena is not present on the subpoena
    D. when the seal of the court is not present on the subpoena

44. A request made to a health information management practitioner by a patient to amend a health record should be referred to
    A. the patient's physician
    B. the hospital's attorney
    C. the hospital administrator
    D. the Chief of Staff

45. All of the following should be part of informed consent for a procedure EXCEPT:
    A. reasonably foreseeable risks of performing the procedure
    B. cost of the procedure
    C. complications or side effects
    D. anticipated results if the procedure is not performed

46. Telephone requests for release of information are best accepted only if
    A. the patient calls personally
    B. the attending physician calls
    C. the patient is under emergency treatment
    D. a physician now treating the patient calls

47. If a physician does not approve of the history and physical report done by a resident, he or she can do any of the following EXCEPT:
    A. remove the history and physical report from the record

B. hand-correct the report

C. add a history and physical of his or her own

D. refuse to countersign the report until the resident corrects it

48. A subpoena duces tecum for a psychiatric record should be
A. complied with
B. refused
C. referred to the Chief of Staff
D. referred to the hospital attorney

49. What is a law called that limits the period of time during which an action may be brought against another party?
A. summons
B. litigation
C. common law
D. statute of limitations

50. Release of information in response to appropriate telephone requests should be made only after
A. the caller's identity is verified
B. contacting the patient
C. contacting the attending physician
D. contacting the hospital administrator

51. Failure to obtain consent to a medical or surgical procedure might result in an action against the physician for
A. battery
B. negligence
C. invasion of privacy
D. intent

52. Defamation includes
A. assault and battery
B. libel and slander
C. negligence and unauthorized disclosure
D. uninformed consent

53. A daily government publication where proposed federal regulations can be found is the
A. *Federal Register*
B. *Common Law Review*
C. *Federal Regulation Register*
D. *Register of Federal Regulation*

54. The medical examiner or coroner would need to provide an authorization to release information from the next of kin or legal representative to perform an autopsy
A. never
B. always
C. only if the deceased were a minor
D. only if death was not a bona fide coroner's case

55. Which of the following could be considered a possible case of negligence?
A. a pedestrian ignores a stranger who is the victim of a hit-and-run driver
B. a hospital patient suffers a broken hip when falling on a wet floor near his room
C. a patient refuses to remain in the hospital, signs forms indicating his consent to release against medical advice, and suffers a heart attack in the hospital's ambulance on the way home
D. a hospital refuses to release a patient until she has arranged for medical insurance to cover her hospital expenses

56. A tort is a wrongful
A. civil act that is not based on a contract violation
B. criminal act involving a health professional and a patient
C. criminal act involving negligence on the part of a physician
D. civil act based on the breaking of an oral contract

57. A person may be required by subpoena to answer questions under oath prior to a trial. This question-and-answer session is called
    A. pretrial discovery
    B. discovery court order
    C. examination before trial
    D. summons

58. The rule that requires that where it is necessary to prove the contents of a paper, the original must be produced or its absence accounted for is called
    A. the best evidence rule
    B. res ipsa loquitur
    C. the judicial notice rule
    D. original evidence

59. The patient, age 17, is to have an appendectomy. He is the son of divorced parents, has been adopted by his grandmother, and is married. Who should sign the operative permit?
    A. wife
    B. grandmother
    C. patient
    D. either parent

60. The term that applies to evidence that may be properly received and considered in a legal proceeding is
    A. best evidence
    B. testimony
    C. demonstrative evidence
    D. admissibility

61. A legal action for unauthorized autopsy in a hospital would be brought against the
    A. hospital pathologist
    B. attending physician
    C. hospital pathologist and the hospital
    D. attending physician and the hospital pathologist

62. In order to verify HIPAA security provisions are met, an organization should have a
    A. Chain-of-Trust Partner Agreement
    B. Business Continuity Plan
    C. Certification of Compliance
    D. Information Access Control Plan

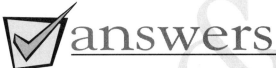

answers & rationales

1.

D. Legally, health records are owned physically by the hospital (Abdelhak, p. 445; Johns, pp. 197, 209).

2.

B. Microfilmed records are considered secondary evidence. However, if the original record is destroyed due to hospital record retention policies and done so in good faith, the microfilmed health record may be used as primary evidence. This is called the best evidence rule (Abdelhak, p. 441; Johns, pp. 771, 786–787).

3.

C. If a patient brings legal action against a physician, the patient automatically gives up the right to confidentiality of information during court proceedings (Abdelhak, pp. 436–437; Johns, p. 193).

4.

D. The hospital's attorney may have immediate access to a patient's records if the patient brings legal action against the facility (Abdelhak, p. 453; Johns, p. 223).

5.

B. Authorizations should be signed by the patient after treatment, so that the patient has better knowledge of what information will be released (Johns, pp. 170–171).

6.

B. The health information technician is not qualified to discuss the diagnosis, treatment, prognosis, or any other medically related questions (Abdelhak, p. 460).

7.

D. Minor errors in typing or spelling may be corrected by writing over the error (Huffman, p. 575).

8.

A. Even though the employer is paying the patient's health insurance or the hospital charges, that fact does not result in a waiver of privileged communication. Only information that would normally be released to an inquirer with a legitimate request and no patient authorization may be given. The patient's prognosis is an item of clinical information and should not be released without proper authorization (Abdelhak, pp. 445–461; Johns, pp. 69–71, 198).

9.

B. The HIM Director should become familiar with state and federal guidelines to make sure he/she responds appropriately to the subpoenas received. The HIM Director must ask the hospital's attorney how to respond to the subpoena, because some states make minutes of medical staff committees inadmissible, others allow the subpoena of such minutes for pretrial discovery purposes, and still others do not address the issue. The server is directed to serve the subpoena to the person named in it (you, as HIM Director), and cannot serve it on anyone else (Abdelhak, pp. 458–460).

10.

B. All of the groups listed in all the answers, except the hospital's Quality Management Committee, should submit a patient authorization or a court order for information about a patient with this diagnosis. The hospital's Quality Management Committee is concerned with the evaluation of medical care provided and, as such, the patient's authorization or a court order is not required (Abdelhak, pp. 454–460).

11.

A. A subpoena requires only that the person named appear. A subpoena duces tecum requires that the person appear with certain specified records. Some jurisdictions allow only the record itself to be sent in response to a subpoena duces tecum. Also, some jurisdictions allow a copy, certified as a true and complete copy of the record, to be sent in response to a subpoena duces tecum (Abdelhak, pp. 453, 458–460; Johns, p. 198).

12.

B. Information from the health record should only be released by the facility that created and owns the record (Abdelhak, pp. 445, 455; Johns, p. 197).

13.

C. If the patient is declared legally incompetent, authorizations may be signed by the person appointed as guardian or legal representative. This person may be the parent or other next of kin (Abdelhak, pp. 223–225).

14.

B. The doctrine of res ipsa loquitur means "the thing speaks for itself." This rule has frequently been applied to two types of malpractice cases: (1) those concerning foreign objects unintentionally left in the body after surgery and (2) injuries to areas of the body that are distant from the site of treatment (Abdelhak, p. 462).

15.

D. This case demonstrates the theory of respondeat superior, which means, "Let the master answer." The employer can be liable for the consequences of employees' actions on the job, whether or not the employer is at fault. Answer A is incorrect, because the hospital medical technologist is not employed by the attending physician but by the hospital. Answer B demonstrates the theory of corporate negligence—even though the attending physician is not employed by the hospital, the hospital may still be considered liable for those working within it. Answer C is incorrect, because the director of nursing services is not the employer of the nurse; she is only her supervisor. The supervisor is also an employee of the hospital and can be held liable only for his or her own actions (Abdelhak, pp. 433, 435).

16.

A. The Supreme Court or the Court of Appeals is the usual name for the final court of appeals at the state level. Other names are the Supreme Court of Errors, Supreme Judicial Court, or Supreme Court of Appeals (Abdelhak, p. 430; Johns, p. 200).

17.

A. Correspondence should be removed, as it does not pertain to the record mentioned in the subpoena (Abdelhak, p. 457).

18.

C. The health record is the property of the hospital. The patient owns the information in the record. The physician has no legal right to the physical record or its information (Abdelhak, p. 445; Johns, p. 197).

19.

C. The incident report and the possibility of its being subpoenaed represent a cloudy issue. One area of agreement is that incident reports are important in studying situations leading to incidents (a function of a risk management program) and that they are less likely to be subpoenaed if a hospital can show that they are specially prepared for the hospital's attorney or insurance carrier. They should never be kept in the health record or the health information management department, because this implies that they are another business record of the hospital and can thus be subpoenaed (Abdelhak, p. 410; Johns, pp. 502–503).

20.

D. The defendant may also be termed the respondent (Abdelhak, p. 432; Johns, p. 201).

21.

A. A minor who is married and economically separated from his parents is considered an emancipated minor and may sign his own authorization. Spouses may not sign authorizations for release of information (Abdelhak, pp. 454–455; Johns, pp. 223–225).

22.

C. Answer A is incorrect because computers can actually improve the completeness, accuracy, and timeliness of health records. Answer B is incorrect because a paper printout of the health record could be produced for use in court. Answer D is incorrect because with Computer Output Microfilm (COM) systems, computer-stored information can be placed directly on microfilm (Abdelhak, pp. 152–158; Johns, pp. 90–91).

23.

B. The standard of care is determined by the jury. The reasonably prudent person is a fictitious, hypothetical character (Abdelhak, pp. 461–462; Johns, p. 202).

24.

A. A person refusing to honor a subpoena can be held in contempt of court. A fine may or may not be imposed as a result (Abdelhak, p. 458; Johns, p. 198).

25.

B. The key factor in retention of records is the state statute of limitations. If there are no specific regulations, or if the facility feels that the statute of limitations is too short, a guideline from the AMA and AHIMA is to keep records for 10 years beyond the most recent episode of care (or if the patient was a minor when treated, 10 years past the age of majority) in either original or microfilm form (Abdelhak, pp. 198–200; Johns, pp. 205–207).

26.

D. Express consent is given after the patient (or an authorized representative) is suitably informed of the treatment to be given, the risks involved, the consequences of treatment, and the alternatives to treatment. Express consent is given directly by the patient, either in writing or verbally. Consent for emergency treatment is implied, since it is assumed that the patient would expressly consent if he or she were able to do so (Abdelhak, p. 91; Johns, p. 65).

27.

B. The physician or surgeon has the responsibility of providing the information necessary to inform the patient adequately before consent is received (Abdelhak, p. 91; Johns, p. 65).

28.

C. An assault is the individual's apprehension of being touched in a way that is insulting, provoking, or injurious without his or her consent. Battery, however, is the actual touching. An assault or battery claim can be made when medical treatment is performed without consent or when an attempt is made to restrain a patient who is competent and oriented without lawful authority (Abdelhak, pp. 433–434).

29.

A. Hearsay evidence, or evidence of a fact based not on the personal observation or knowledge of the witness but on what someone else said, is not admissible as evidence. Hearsay evidence can be oral or written. One exception to the hearsay rule is the business records rule, which allows records kept in the regular course of a business or professional activity (including hospital or physician records) to be admitted as evidence. The extent to which the business records rule acts as an exception to the hearsay rule is a matter for court decision or statute in individual states (Abdelhak, p. 441).

30.

C. The bill of particulars in a civil action is an itemized or detailed account of the matters set forth in the pleading (which consists of the written allegations of the plaintiff and defendant, consisting of the plaintiff's complaint and the defendant's answer) (Abdelhak, p. 432; Johns, pp. 201–202).

31.

B. A court of original jurisdiction is one in which cases and special proceedings are tried. Courts of appellate jurisdiction hear appeals from courts of original jurisdiction (Abdelhak, pp. 430–432; Johns, p. 200).

32.

A. The patient in essence owns the information in the record and has the right to control its release (Abdelhak, p. 445; Johns, p. 197).

33.

B. Although the health information management department cannot control the redisclosure of information it has released, it is helpful to include a statement prohibiting the redisclosure with any released information (Abdelhak, pp. 456–457).

34.

B. An attorney may issue a subpoena, signing it personally, and attest it in the name of a judge, a court, the clerk, or another proper officer. It need not be countersigned and it cannot be ignored (Abdelhak, pp. 453–460; Johns, p. 198).

35.

D. The plaintiff may also be called the petitioner, complainant, or declarant (Abdelhak, p. 432; Johns, p. 201).

36.

D. This term was invented by the authors (Abdelhak, pp. 447–450; Johns, pp. 223–224).

37.

D. No information at all, even the fact that the patient was seen for treatment, can be released by any health care facility with an identified unit set aside for treating patients with alcohol abuse (Abdelhak, p. 443; Johns, p. 70).

38.

D. The attending physician needs to be notified only if there is a possibility that the record will be involved in a malpractice suit. The administrator should also be notified in this case (Abdelhak, pp. 432–433; Johns, p. 508).

39.

A. The signature of the individual requesting information is not necessary because the authorization comes from the patient (or his or her representative) and should bear his or her signature. The other items, along with others specified in the reference given, should be included. The student should be familiar with items considered necessary for a proper written authorization (Abdelhak, pp. 444–450; Johns, p. 69).

40.

D. Some states, however, allow minors to seek treatment for certain conditions without the consent of their parent or legal guardian. In such cases, the parent or legal guardian cannot authorize release of information (Abdelhak, pp. 454–455).

41.

A. The privilege belongs to the patient, enabling him or her to feel secure in disclosing information. Only the patient can normally relinquish the privilege (Johns, p. 202).

42.

D. Financial data are not medical information (Abdelhak, p. 77; Johns, p. 136).

43.

A. The signature of the patient (who might not even be bringing or defending a legal action at all—there might be a suit pending between two automobile insurance companies, for example) is not required.

The other items should be included in a subpoena. A subpoena lacking these items is invalid and does not have to be accepted. The attorney who caused the subpoena to be issued should be notified (Abdelhak, p. 453; Johns, p. 198).

44.

A. If the physician concurs with the patient's request, hospital policy should describe how the record should be amended (Abdelhak, p. 103).

45.

B. Although the cost of the procedure is of interest, it is not considered information required for legally informed consent (Abdelhak, pp. 462–464; Johns, p. 65).

46.

C. All other requests are better handled in writing in order to better protect the hospital and the patient (Abdelhak, p. 447).

47.

A. Any removal of reports from a record may suggest that an effort is being made to suppress evidence because of the business records rule, which allows records kept in the regular course of a business or professional activity (including hospital or physician records) to be admitted as evidence. The extent to which the business records rule acts as an exception to the hearsay rule is a matter for court decision or statute in individual states (Abdelhak, p. 441).

48.

A. Psychiatric records are no more privileged than any other record arising out of the physician–patient relationship; a subpoena duces tecum for psychiatric records should be treated in the same way as for any other records (Abdelhak, p. 453).

49.

D. Statutes of limitations establish the time limit within which lawsuits can be brought (Abdelhak, p. 438).

50.

A. The usual method of verifying the caller's identity is to offer to call back. Since a telephone response is normally made only in response to other health care providers treating the patient, verification of identity can be made by checking the telephone book, telephone information, or by the response of the person answering the call back (Huffman, p. 589).

51.

A. Battery is unlawful touching (Abdelhak, p. 433).

52.

B. Libel is the written form and slander is the verbal form of defamation or false statements that tend to injure character or reputation (Abdelhak, p. 434).

53.

A. Interested persons can respond to proposed regulations or changes to existing regulations by writing to the agency proposing the regulation. Final regulations are also published in the *Federal Register.* The other answers are fabrications (Abdelhak, p. 378).

54.

D. If the case is considered a coroner's case (e.g., a homicide, suicide, etc.) an authorization for release of information for autopsy is not required from the next of kin or legal representative (Abdelhak, p. 454).

55.

B. The hospital should have foreseen that the wet floor could cause harm, and the magnitude of the risk was such that the hospital should have provided a safer environment (Abdelhak, pp. 461–462).

56.

A. A tort is a wrongful civil act that is not based on a violation of a contract (Abdelhak, p. 428; Johns, p. 202).

57.

C. Pretrial discovery is the process whereby one side in a lawsuit can obtain information possessed by others, either by examining the other side or his or her witnesses or by examination of documents. The most frequently used discovery court orders are subpoenas. During an examination before trial, the deposition, or sworn statement, of a person is taken; if the person cannot later attend the trial, the deposition can be used as his or her testimony. A summons is an order to appear before the court (Abdelhak, p. 432; Johns, p. 201).

58.

A. The best evidence rule requires that the original health record be produced in court. Most jurisdictions now allow a certified copy of the record to be produced, or a microfilm if the original record has been microfilmed (Abdelhak, p. 441).

59.

C. This individual is an emancipated minor because he is married, and he can sign his own consent for surgery. If he were not married, his grandmother, as legal guardian, would need to sign the consent (Abdelhak, p. 455).

60.

D. Admissible evidence is any evidence that is relevant to the case, is competent, and tends to support either the plaintiff's complaint or the defendant's defense (Abdelhak, p. 432).

61.

C. Even though salaried by the hospital, the pathologist can be held liable. The hospital is also held liable because hospital autopsies are done at the direction of the hospital administration (Abdelhak, pp. 433, 465).

62.

C. The Certification of Compliance is a good way to verify the organization meets the security criteria set forth by HIPAA. The Chain-of-Trust Agreement is a signed contract between healthcare facilities and third parties to ensure data integrity and confidentiality. A Business Continuity Plan is a plan set for natural disasters that may shut down the computer system. Information Access Control Plan is a made-up term. Information Access Controls are policies and procedures set forth to allow different levels of access to the computer system (Johns, p. 674).

8 Information Technology

objectives

After completion of this chapter, the student will be able to:

➤ Explain the evolution of health care information systems.

➤ Define computer software utilized in health care including application software, hardware, programming languages, and networks.

➤ Describe computer networks utilized in the health care field.

➤ List the steps and different plans associated with information systems planning.

➤ Discuss the systems development life cycle.

➤ Differentiate between data versus information.

➤ Identify data integrity and security.

➤ Provide examples of administrative, HIM, and clinical health information systems utilized in the health care field.

➤ Explain the technological advances in the HIM field.

DIRECTIONS (Questions 1–67): Each of the questions or incomplete statements below is followed by suggested answers or completions. Select the **best** answer in each case.

1. In order to be useful, data must be
   A. collated
   B. arranged
   C. processed
   D. filed

2. In designing a new information system, the primary consideration should be the
   A. cost of the system
   B. requirements of the users
   C. available technology
   D. space available to house the system

3. One disadvantage of dedicated word processing systems is
   A. they cannot store large numbers of documents
   B. their cost is very high
   C. they can only be used for word processing
   D. they break down frequently

4. Which of the following is not considered a way to improve the security of data in a computerized MPI?
   A. audit trail
   B. user password
   C. increasing the number of users
   D. policies and procedures

5. Major hardware components of many telecommunications systems are
   A. cables
   B. modems
   C. CD-ROM drives
   D. telegraph wires

6. Electronic mail is an example of a data communications application called
   A. message switching
   B. remote job entry
   C. source data collection
   D. time-sharing

7. Information is
   A. less complex than data
   B. part of data
   C. more complex than data
   D. compiled from data

8. An integrated group of related activities that work together toward a common goal is a
   A. system
   B. supersystem
   C. set
   D. mission

9. A hardware device that data may be entered into or retrieved from is
   A. storage
   B. control unit
   C. arithmetic/logic unit
   D. input device

10. The portion of the computer that directs the sequence of operations, interprets the coded instructions (the program), and initiates the proper commands to the computer circuits is the
    A. storage
    B. control unit
    C. arithmetic/logic unit
    D. peripheral unit

11. Careful planning to ensure that all required components exist in an information system, including appropriate equipment and programs, is generally encompassed in
    A. profile analysis

B. the data processing cycle

C. systems analysis

D. computer analysis

12. The concept of multiple users for one computer is termed
   A. multiuser facility
   B. time-sharing
   C. real-time operation
   D. facility sharing

13. In microcomputers, the primary input device is the
   A. CPU
   B. monitor
   C. keyboard
   D. cable

14. Ethernet is an example of
   A. network topology
   B. WAN
   C. token ring
   D. star network

15. Which of the following is not considered a basic element of the data processing cycle?
   A. output
   B. storage
   C. input
   D. control unit

16. A problem with traditional manual file systems is that the same data are often stored in many different places. This is termed
   A. data representation
   B. data redundancy
   C. data flow
   D. data design

17. A kilobyte is equal to
   A. 512 characters
   B. 1 million characters

C. 1,024 characters

D. 1/1,000 of a character

18. In designing a record tracking system, all of the following are facts that would most probably best be supplied by the health information management director EXCEPT:
   A. the number of medical records on file
   B. the number of locations the medical records might be used in the facility
   C. the duration of time medical records may spend in one location
   D. the costs of various components of the system

19. A system that shows who has accessed what information in a computer system, such as a patient registration database, is called a (an)
   A. audit trail
   B. smart card
   C. voiceprint
   D. password

20. The most sophisticated application of computers is
   A. word processing
   B. graphics
   C. windowing programs
   D. artificial intelligence

21. Client-server technology is comprised of
   A. a host computer and several workstations
   B. a network of personal computers with equal functionality
   C. a mainframe and several dumb terminals
   D. a standalone personal computer

22. All of the following can be used to connect computers together in a network EXCEPT:
   A. twisted pair wiring
   B. fiber optic cabling
   C. telephone wiring
   D. modems

23. In dictation systems, recording media that can be physically removed from the dictation equipment are termed
    A. discrete
    B. discontinuous
    C. partial
    D. handheld

24. Assume that one page of copy will hold 250 words. How many kilobytes of storage will be needed to store one page (one word equals six characters)?
    A. 1.75
    B. 1,500
    C. 4.10
    D. 1.46

25. A bedside terminal might use any of the following input devices EXCEPT:
    A. light pen
    B. keyboard
    C. touch screen
    D. digital plotter

26. Applications in which word processing may be useful include all of the following EXCEPT:
    A. tumor or cancer registry
    B. birth certificates
    C. budget
    D. medical staff committee minutes

27. One of the greatest challenges of computerizing health information is
    A. system breakdown
    B. confidentiality
    C. cost of obtaining new systems
    D. maintenance cost

28. A device used in telecommunications, using telephone wires, is a
    A. modem
    B. printer
    C. network
    D. plotter

29. An optical disk storage system can store medical information from any of the following sources EXCEPT:
    A. paper reports
    B. radiologic images
    C. text transcribed using a word processor
    D. subpoenae duces tecum

30. The part of a computer system that contains instructions for storing, manipulating, and retrieving data is termed the
    A. control unit
    B. storage unit
    C. program
    D. arithmetic/logic unit

31. The industry standard for the average business word is five characters plus a space. How many words can be stored in a kilobyte of memory?
    A. 170
    B. 1,024
    C. 124
    D. 512

32. In an optical disk storage system, jukeboxes store
    A. optical disk platters
    B. optical disk software
    C. printers
    D. reports

33. An example of a high-level computer language is
    A. machine language
    B. MUMPS
    C. DOS
    D. assembly language

34. "The process of connecting records on the same individual that have been generated at different times and in different places" is called
   A. record analysis
   B. record linkage
   C. data linkage
   D. information analysis

35. A system whereby several microcomputers within a small geographic area are linked is called a
   A. ring formation
   B. star network
   C. wide area network
   D. local area network

36. Discrete storage media in a centralized dictation system using a telephone network include all of the following EXCEPT:
   A. plastic belts or disks
   B. microcassettes
   C. magnetic belts
   D. endless loop magnetic tape

37. The process of entering every medication provided, diagnostic test performed, meal served, and other patient service into a system is called
   A. cost accounting
   B. case-mix analysis
   C. charge capture
   D. claims processing

38. Medicare inpatient claims are submitted using the
   A. HCFA-1500
   B. UB-92
   C. accounts receivable
   D. ECMS

39. All of the following are output devices EXCEPT:
   A. optical character readers
   B. microfilm units
   C. audio response devices
   D. printers

40. Computer-generated information regarding patient accounts not yet paid could assist the health information management department in all of the following EXCEPT:
   A. determining which health records are not yet filed in the permanent file
   B. determining which health records are not yet received from the nursing units
   C. determining which health records are not yet coded
   D. determining which health records have not yet had abstracted data entered into the computer system that provides information for billing purposes

41. A computerized Registration-Admissions, Discharges and Transfers (R-ADT) system would be used by
   A. the health information management department
   B. the admitting department
   C. the billing department
   D. several departments, including the health information management department

42. Peripheral devices include
   A. input–output devices
   B. control unit
   C. primary memory
   D. software

43. Computer systems can aid nursing management in all of the following ways EXCEPT:
   A. determining patient acuity levels
   B. automation of practice guidelines
   C. providing counseling to nursing personnel
   D. scheduling nursing personnel

44. An example of self-contained dictation media is a
    A. tank
    B. cassette
    C. disk
    D. roll

45. A disadvantage of a shared resource type of word processing system over a standalone system is that
    A. only one person may use the system at any one time
    B. it is the most costly type of system
    C. when the system is down, no users are able to work with it
    D. media storage is less efficient

46. A health information management department manager would most likely use spreadsheet software for
    A. budgeting
    B. fi-360 chart tracking
    C. correspondence control
    D. tumor registry

47. The application whereby a physician enters a request for a particular laboratory test and is able to review the outcome is called
    A. test entry/outcome reporting
    B. laboratory entry/results review
    C. test data entry/laboratory results reporting
    D. order entry/results reporting

48. Computer-based repositories of knowledge are called
    A. text-based systems
    B. expert systems
    C. library systems
    D. alert systems

49. Controls that can improve the accuracy of data in a computerized health information system must be able to assist all of the following EXCEPT:
    A. error detection
    B. error location
    C. error manipulation
    D. error correction

50. All of the following are examples of administrative information systems that support the daily management of healthcare facilities EXCEPT:
    A. patient registration systems
    B. financial information systems
    C. human resource management systems
    D. clinical decision support systems

51. _____ are attached to databases for the purpose of diverting the transmission of data.
    A. sniffers
    B. hackers
    C. both B and C
    D. none of the above

52. Which of the following is not a subcategory of the management support system, which provides reporting information?
    A. management information systems
    B. strategic decision support systems
    C. facilities management systems
    D. executive information systems

53. HIPAA data security provisions are divided into four sections, which include administrative provisions, physical safeguards, technical safeguards, and _____.
    A. personnel
    B. environmental
    C. network and communication
    D. none of the above

54. The systems development life cycle (SDLC) includes four general phases that follow what sequence?
    A. design, planning and analysis, implementation, maintenance and evaluation

B. planning and analysis, design, implementation, maintenance and evaluation

C. planning and analysis, implementation, maintenance and evaluation, design

D. design, implementation, planning and implementation, maintenance and evaluation

55. What type of communication device is used for patients to access information regarding office locations or patient educational materials?

A. information kiosk

B. Web center

C. E-mail communication

D. Smart card

56. As project manager of a new computer-based system at your healthcare facility, you are at the point where you must create the request for proposal. What phase of the systems development life cycle are you in?

A. planning and analysis

B. design

C. implementation

D. maintenance and evaluation

57. Who is responsible for leading the strategic IS planning process for assisting and overseeing the organizations IS functions?

A. Chief Information Officer (CIO)

B. Information Systems Steering Committee

C. Chief Security Officer (CSO)

D. Chief Privacy Officer

58. A physician at your hospital wants to check on a patient and logs on to the computer where he/she looks at the patient's status, laboratory results, recent medications given, and former history and physical information. The software that can converge different types of documents together to allow this process is called

A. videoconferencing

B. groupware

C. decision support systems

D. interactive voice technology

59. The term _____ controls refer to the implementation of procedures used to keep documented logs of system access and access attempts with regards to HIPAA standards.

A. physical access

B. audit

C. authorization

D. access

60. The standard user interface that uses icons that represent different computer tasks and programs is known as

A. programming languages

B. structured query language (SQL)

C. graphical user interface (GUI)

D. database management system (DBMS)

61. Public Law 104-191, passed in 1996, which provides data security practices and standards, is known as the

A. Centers for Medicare and Medicaid Services (CMS)

B. Health Insurance Portability and Accountability Act (HIPAA)

C. National Research Council 2000 (NRC)

D. Computer-based Patient Record Institute (CPRI)

62. You are a HIM Director and are in the process of writing a request for proposal (RFP) for a new system. The vendors that you have selected to complete the cost–benefit analysis are Oracle, SQL Server, Sybase, and Access. What type of information system are you researching?

A. spreadsheet system

B. word processing system

C. database management system

D. graphical presentation system

63. What is the common language that is used to store and retrieve data in any database management system?

    A. use of ones and zeros (binary language)
    B. standard set of abbreviations
    C. COBOL and BASIC
    D. structured query language (SQL)

64. What type of database stores data in pre-defined tables made up of rows and columns?

    A. relational database
    B. object-oriented database
    C. object-relational database
    D. none of the above

65. Computer networks rely on _____ that use the same language to communicate.

    A. controls
    B. servers
    C. protocols
    D. services

66. Data _____ provides the ability of a business to access data from multiple databases and combine the results into a single reporting interface.

    A. dictionary
    B. warehouse
    C. security
    D. availability

67. _____ encodes information and converts it to unreadable symbols and characters, which must be decoded for the purpose of protecting data.

    A. Access controls
    B. Authorization controls
    C. Encryption
    D. Entity authentication

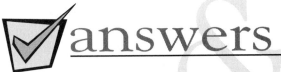

answers & rationales

1.

C. Data alone do not have much purpose until they have been interpreted in some way. They then become information (Abdelhak, p. 77; Johns, p. 23).

2.

B. The needs of the users of any system must be analyzed first, because a computer system may not even be necessary to meet these needs. Once the necessity of having a system is established, other criteria (including those given in answers A, C, and D) can be considered (Abdelhak, p. 722).

3.

C. If other functions are required (e.g., database, spreadsheet, a chart location system), then a computer capable of running these functions might be better. Costs, downtime, and storage capabilities can be the same or quite different (Abdelhak, p. 446; Johns, pp. 596–599).

4.

C. As more users access the master patient index, the risk of a security breach increases; the other three answers help reduce this risk (Abdelhak, pp. 153, 157, 186–188).

5.

B. Modems allow the computer to receive and transmit data over telephone lines (Abdelhak, p. 681).

6.

A. Message switching permits the sending of a message from one terminal to another (Johns, p. 128).

7.

C. Data alone do not have much purpose until they have been interpreted in some way. They then become information (Abdelhak, p. 77; Johns, p. 23).

8.

A. The health facility is itself a system. The computerization that supports the functions of the health facility is also a system (Abdelhak, p. 537).

9.

A. Storage or memory holds data until needed. The control unit directs data to and from the arithmetic/logic unit. All three of these components make up the central processing unit, or CPU. An input device is a means to enter data into the CPU (Abdelhak, p. 168; Johns, pp. 607–608).

10.

B. Storage or memory holds data until needed. The control unit directs data to and from the arithmetic/logic unit. All three of these components (storage, control unit, and arithmetic/logic unit) make up the central processing unit, or CPU (Abdelhak, p. 168; Johns, pp. 607–608).

11.

C. A thorough discussion of systems analysis is given in Abdelhak (pp. 729–747).

12.

B. Time-sharing allows small information systems to use large computer installations by leasing time and sharing the facilities with many other users (Abdelhak, p. 505).

13.

C. An input device is used to feed data into the computer. A mouse or other pointing device may be used as an adjunct to a keyboard (Abdelhak, p. 169; Johns, pp. 607–608).

14.

A. Ethernet and token ring are topologies or patterns for wiring users together in a Local Area Network (LAN). They are communication protocols or rules used in a network configuration. A WAN or Wide Area Network is a geographically disbursed group of users (Abdelhak, pp. 174, 665; Johns, p. 620).

15.

D. The control unit is part of the CPU (hardware). Other basic elements of the data processing cycle include data origination (source documents) and manipulation (processing) (Johns, pp. 607–608).

16.

B. Computer database software helps solve the problem of data redundancy (Abdelhak, pp. 148–149).

17.

C. A megabyte (or MB) is approximately 1 million bytes (Freedman, p. 101).

18.

D. Information on costs probably would be supplied by system manufacturers or systems analysts, either the hospital's own personnel or consultants hired by the hospital (Abdelhak, p. 722).

19.

A. The audit trail can show activities of people or equipment used (e.g., a computer terminal used after a department has closed for the day) (Abdelhak, p. 157; Johns, p. 671).

20.

D. Artificial intelligence is a special type of computer programming in which software models are used to handle functions that would require the intellectual capabilities of humans (Johns, p. 611).

21.

A. The host is the server—it is usually more powerful than the client workstation. The client handles as many functions as possible to reduce server processing time. The server performs functions that the clients cannot, such as database and network management and security functions (Abdelhak, p. 174; Johns, pp. 616, 619).

22.

D. Modems are the hardware components that allow the computer to use telephone wiring to carry data to and from other computers. Twisted pair and fiber optic cabling are two examples of direct wiring among computers in a network (Abdelhak, pp. 665–666).

23.

A. Discrete media include cassettes, minicassettes, microcassettes, belts, and disks (Johns, pp. 772–773).

24.

D. First, multiply 250 words by 6 characters per word = 1,500 characters on the page. Because a kilobyte stores 1,024 characters, the next step is to divide the number of characters on the page (1,500) by 1,024 to get 1.464 (Abdelhak, p. 146).

25.

D. Digital plotters are specialized printers, output devices (Abdelhak, pp. 201–204; Johns, p. 608).

26.

C. A spreadsheet application would be better to computerize a budget (Abdelhak, pp. 661–662).

27.

B. One way of securing confidentiality is through built-in levels of information: Certain levels can only be accessed through secret codes or passwords. Other ways are through plastic cards identifying the user, or using computer output that is encrypted and needs special software to be unscrambled (Abdelhak, pp. 677–682; Johns, pp. 162, 679).

28.

A. Printers and plotters (a specialized form of printer) are connected directly to a computer via cable. A network may include computers that are connected by modem or cable (Abdelhak, p. 681).

29.

D. This is so only because subpoenas do not contain medical information (Abdelhak, pp. 216–217).

30.

C. The program, or parts of it, is used by all parts of the CPU (answers A, B, and D) (Abdelhak, pp. 173–174; Johns, p. 611).

31.

A. A kilobyte stores 1,024 characters. A business word equals five characters plus a space, which is also a character, for a total of six characters. The answer is found by dividing: $1{,}024 \div 6 = 170.66$. An argument can be made that the correct answer should be rounded to 171; on the other hand, that extra six characters would not fit in the kilobyte. Therefore, the answer is rounded down to 170 (Freedman, p. 526).

32.

A. The jukebox is a library of platters (Abdelhak, p. 217).

33.

A. Others include FORTRAN, PASCAL, and BASIC. Operating system software (DOS is an example) is commonly written using assembly language (Abdelhak, p. 173; Johns, p. 611).

34.

B. The computer makes record linkage in health care more feasible (Abdelhak, p. 45).

35.

D. See Abdelhak, pp. 204–205, for a discussion of the other three terms (see also Johns, p. 620).

36.

D. Endless loop magnetic tape is an example of self-contained media (Johns, pp. 772–773).

37.

C. Capturing all charges gives both providers and payors more accurate information on resources used to treat patients (Abdelhak, p. 625).

38.

B. Accounts receivable are accounts for which the hospital is waiting to receive payment. ECMS (electronic medical claims submission) is the process of transmitting medical claims via data communications technology (Abdelhak, p. 235; Johns, p. 385).

39.

A. Other output devices include visual display devices and digital plotters (Abdelhak, pp. 201–204; Johns, p. 608).

40.

A. Because accounts receivable are accounts not yet paid (and perhaps not yet billed), the list of cases on such a report can help determine which cases have not yet been received, coded, or abstracted (Abdelhak, p. 625).

41.

D. The R-ADT system is an interdepartmental system that can be used by most departments in the health facility, although these systems are typically under the control of the admitting or patient registration department. The system provides a central database on the health facility's patients (Abdelhak, p. 697).

42.

A. A peripheral device is hardware other than the CPU. Primary storage or memory is contained within the CPU. Software is not a hardware device (Abdelhak, pp. 168–169; Johns, pp. 607–608).

43.

A. Computer systems and new technology can enhance and improve quality of patient care services (Johns, pp. 686–687).

44.

A. Self-contained media are not physically handled, as are discrete media such as cassettes or disks. Rolls (answer D) concern microfilm rather than dictation equipment (Johns, pp. 772–773).

45.

C. Answer A is the major disadvantage of a standalone system. Answer B may or may not be true. Efficient media storage is an advantage of shared systems (Abdelhak, pp. 59–60).

46.

A. Spreadsheets are used for budgeting purposes (Abdelhak, pp. 661–662; Johns, p. 610).

47.

A. Such systems greatly facilitate the transmittal of physician orders and the speed of receiving results (Johns, p. 648).

48.

A. Such systems include knowledge of experts in the particular area of interest. Two parts to expert medical systems are online searching for medical information and computer-aided diagnosis and treatment (Abdelhak, pp. 671–672; Johns, p. 598).

49.

A. This answer is fabricated. Abdelhak provides a discussion of the other three answers (pp. 166–167).

50.

D. Is an example of a patient care and department clinical system. Answers A, B, and C represent the management-related operations of a health care facility (Johns, p. 567).

51.

A. Sniffers divert information when data is transmitted; thus, encryption is utilized to minimize the threat of security threats. Sniffers are known to "eavesdrop" on the transmission of data. Hackers try to break into systems for the purpose of obtaining and/or manipulating password and confidential information (Johns, p. 679).

52.

C. An example of a MIS report would be daily hospital census. An example of a strategic decision support system would be reports to evaluate performance indicators and trends. An example of an executive information system report would be yearly length-of-stay statistics (Johns, pp. 568–569).

53.

C. HIPAA data security provisions include administrative, physical, technical, and network and communication safeguards to minimize the threat of security breach (Johns, p. 673).

54.

B. The systems development life cycle is an ongoing process that goes through the planning and analysis, design, implementation and maintenance, and evaluation (Johns, pp. 572–573).

55.

A. Kiosks are computer stations set up for patient access in health care facilities to provide information about the facility, that is, locations (Johns, p. 616).

56.

B. During the design phase, systems available on the market and the vendor selection process takes place along with the request for proposal (RFP), which is a detailed description of the requirements for the system, cost–benefit analysis, and contract negotiations (Johns, pp. 572–575).

57.

A. The CIO is a senior-level executive who oversees the organization's IS functions. The IS steering committee's role is to determine the strategic vision of the information systems for the organization, which include clinicians, administrators, etc. The CSO is responsible for overseeing the development, implementation, and enforcement of the organization's security policies. The Chief Privacy Officer's role is to oversee policies and procedures relating to privacy and access of patient information (Johns, pp. 581–582).

58.

B. Groupware is a application software program used by physicians that allow the physician to look at different documents on the program simultaneously, such as history and physicals, laboratory results, medication records, progress notes, etc. Videoconferencing is used to connect people from different locations to communicate in one room during a meeting. Decision support systems are used by clinicians to make decisions about the patient's diagnosis and treatment plan. Interactive voice technology allows the user to call an automated system to retrieve patient information, that is, X-ray results (Johns, pp. 690, 696–697).

59.

B. Audit controls are utilized to keep track of who is accessing and attempting to access data in a healthcare facility (Johns, pp. 677–678).

60.

(C) The GUI allows for the pointing and clicking of the mouse on the icons that represent a computer function (Johns, p. 610).

61.

B. HIPAA was enacted in 1996, which provided standards for security of health information on a national level (Johns, pp. 662–663, 673).

62.

C. The different kinds of database management system vendors on the market would be those listed in the question (Johns, p. 612).

63.

D. SQL includes a query language to generate reports (Johns, p. 611).

64.

A. The relational database stores predefined tables that contain columns and rows that look like a spreadsheet. An object database stores objects of data (Johns, p. 612).

65.

C. According to Johns, "Network protocols enable computers on the network to communicate with each other" (p. 620).

66.

B. A data warehouse allows an organization to manipulate data from different databases and to combine the results into a single interface. A data dictionary is a list of data elements for an information system. Data security refers to keeping data safe from tampering. Data availability refers to information being accessible at any point (Johns, pp. 616–617).

67.

C. The use of encryption converts text into unreadable information and the text must be decoded. This allows for the highest level of data security (Johns, p. 679).

9 Quality Assessment and Performance Improvement

objectives

After completion of this chapter, the student will be able to:

➤ Explain QI collection tools, data analysis, and reporting techniques utilized in the health care field.

➤ Describe Utilization Management and its role in the quality assessment and improvement process.

➤ Identify the QI pioneers and their respective philosophies.

➤ Determine the appropriate uses of methods to display data to assist in quality assessment.

➤ Discuss Risk Management and its role in the quality assessment and imrovement process.

➤ Explain clinical pathways and case management.

➤ Summarize the accreditation and licensing quality improvement standards in the health care field.

DIRECTIONS (Questions 1–66): Each of the questions or incomplete statements below is followed by suggested answers or completions. Select the **best** answer in each case.

1. A transcription unit has six transcriptionists, two of whom work half time. If their average production is as given in the following table, what is the average output per FTE (in lines per day)?

Transcriptionist	Lines/Day
A	950
B	450
C	600
D	1,100
E	1,050
F	1,000

   A. 1,033 lines per day
   B. 1,030 lines per day
   C. 858 lines per day
   D. 5,150 lines per day

2. Quality management includes all of the following EXCEPT:
   A. risk management
   B. quality assessment
   C. utilization management
   D. billing process review

3. A hospital's utilization management plan should outline all of the following EXCEPT:
   A. the organization of the committee
   B. the administrative support for the utilization management program
   C. the relationship of the utilization management program to other quality management activities
   D. qualifications of the utilization management coordinator

4. Programs designed to control liability for human errors and equipment failures are termed
   A. utilization review/management programs

   B. quality management programs
   C. risk management programs
   D. continuing education programs

5. Which type of review is not considered a medical staff function included in the quality management program?
   A. blood usage review
   B. medical record review
   C. surgical case review
   D. safety review

6. To develop a frame of reference in order to understand the major facts, issues, and underlying theories already addressed that surround the research topic, the researcher should not do which of the following?
   A. review literature in his or her own discipline
   B. review literature in other disciplines
   C. ignore if no literature in one's discipline is available
   D. consult with colleagues and/or experts

7. Once the problem is found to be a feasible topic for study and has been clearly formulated, a second literature review at this point
   A. is not necessary
   B. can be minimal
   C. is more selective than the first review
   D. is unhelpful in determining the research design

8. A health information management's transcription unit is open Monday through Friday during the day. It is responsible for transcribing an average of 200,000 lines of dictation in each 4-week period. The transcription minimum productivity standard for this unit

is 1,000 lines per day. How many FTE (full-time equivalent) transcriptionists are needed to staff the unit?

A. 10.0
B. 7.14
C. 40.0
D. 8.0

9. PL 92-603 provided for the establishment of
   A. PSROs
   B. JCAHO as a government organization
   C. PROs
   D. ACS

10. Risk management programs were introduced to reduce
    A. hospital charges
    B. malpractice suits
    C. the number of hospital personnel
    D. complaints related to billing

11. Screening criteria used in utilization review must be
    A. objective
    B. subjective
    C. approved by the quality management committee
    D. written by the individuals to whose services the criteria will be applied

12. Utilization review/management (UR/UM) first became mandatory
    A. with the passage of Medicare legislation
    B. with the passage of PSRO legislation
    C. when JCAHO assumed the task of accrediting hospitals
    D. as each state passed UR legislation

13. The QI pioneer who developed the three-faceted approach to quality or quality triangle, which included the quality, all-one-team, scientific approach.

A. W. Edward Deming
B. Joseph Juran
C. Philip Crosby
D. Brian Joiner

14. The process advocated by JCAHO to monitor, evaluate, and solve problems in patient care is called the
    A. JCAHO process
    B. 10-step process
    C. Medicare Quality Management process
    D. clinical monitoring and evaluation process

15. PL 92-603 was
    A. an amendment to the Social Security Act
    B. the law establishing risk management programs in hospitals
    C. the law establishing quality management programs in hospitals
    D. the law that established the Medicare program

16. Once a patient care service defines its important aspects of care, which of the following does not occur?
    A. indicators are developed
    B. the service's major functions are defined
    C. thresholds are defined
    D. indicators are evaluated

17. Under PL 92-603, all hospitals were required to have a
    A. UR (UM) coordinator
    B. UR (UM) department
    C. UR (UM) secretary
    D. UR (UM) plan

18. Incident reports are analyzed
    A. concurrently
    B. within 1 month of discharge
    C. immediately after discharge
    D. within 3 months of discharge

19. A transcription unit supervisor decides that an error rate of 2% or less is acceptable; in other words, no more than 2% of the lines typed may contain errors. Through proof-reading a sample of work, it is found that there are 156 lines with errors among 2,586 lines of dictation. This unit has
    A. exactly met its standard
    B. done better than its standard
    C. done worse than its standard
    D. an error rate that cannot be calculated, given the information provided

20. As a result of external pressure to contain costs, many hospitals are entering into insurance plans that provide clients (i.e., patients) with incentives to use that particular hospital. Such plans are termed
    A. health maintenance organizations
    B. preferred provider organizations
    C. fixed-cost associations
    D. community health provider organizations

21. The purposes of QIOs does not include determining which of the following?
    A. whether services provided were medically necessary
    B. whether the quality of services provided met professionally recognized standards of health care
    C. whether the care was provided in the most economical setting consistent with the patient's health care needs
    D. whether the health care facility had met accreditation and licensing standards

22. A tool for identifying potential risks before an incident occurs is the
    A. hazard surveillance report
    B. quality assessment report
    C. risk management report
    D. utilization management report

23. In 1986, JCAHO launched a major new quality project that was intended to shift its emphasis from review of structure and process to review of
    A. risk reduction
    B. outcome
    C. credentialing
    D. utilization review procedures

24. Relevant findings from quality management activities must be considered as part of the
    A. reappointment of medical staff members
    B. selection or election of medical staff officers
    C. renewal of contracts with hospital counsel
    D. renewal of contracts with third-party payors

25. The type of review not performed in the UR/UM process is which of the following?
    A. concurrent review
    B. applied review
    C. retrospective review
    D. preadmission review

26. If the need for admission cannot be determined, the case is first referred to
    A. the attending physician
    B. a physician reviewer
    C. the utilization management coordinator
    D. the Utilization Management Committee

27. A mechanism that can help identify risk from physician-related activities is termed
    A. quality screening
    B. incident screening
    C. hazard screening
    D. occurrence screening

28. A stringent test of the quality of professional research is
    A. its ability to be duplicated with the same results

B. whether the results agree with the hypothesis

C. whether the research project can be completed

D. whether funding can be obtained to complete the research project

29. Which of the following would not be considered an example of overutilization?

A. repeated tests due to delays in reporting of results

B. premature discharge

C. ancillary services that are not beneficial

D. ambulatory care provided to an inpatient

30. The primary tool for identifying risk is the

A. medical record

B. incident report

C. subpoena duces tecum

D. diagnostic index

31. Besides JCAHO, organization(s) that strongly influence(s) quality management activity in a hospital is (are)

A. Medicare

B. Centers for Disease Control

C. state cancer registries

D. medical specialty boards

32. An example of hospitalwide quality assessment is

A. credentialing

B. blood usage review

C. dietetic review

D. infection control

33. Which of the following is not considered an example of research design?

A. descriptive studies

B. featured studies

C. exploratory studies

D. testing of causal relationships

34. Two types of causal research design are

A. comparative and correlational

B. historical and exploratory

C. survey and investigative

D. descriptive and experimental

35. Which of the following is not a data-gathering method?

A. measurement

B. observation

C. correlation

D. questioning

36. If you want to analyze the relationship between age and weight in female patients over age 30, which diagram would help you determine if there is a relationship or not?

A. run chart

B. scatter diagram

C. pareto chart

D. flow chart

37. The sampling technique that is used when, for example, every 10th member of the population is chosen, is called

A. simple random

B. stratified random

C. cluster

D. systematic

38. An HIM department might utilize this QI tool to chart trends in response time to physicians' record requests

A. histogram

B. bar graph

C. frequency polygon

D. comparative list

39. This QI pioneer believed that the standard for quality should be "zero defects."

A. W. Edward Deming

B. Joseph Juran

C. Philip Crosby

D. Brian Joiner

40. The measure that shows the degree to which scores scatter around the mean is called the
    A. median
    B. t-score
    C. variance
    D. z-score

41. When a researcher rejects the null hypothesis when it is true, the error is called
    A. a type II error
    B. a statistical error
    C. an error in significance
    D. a type I error

42. The exact reverse of the research hypothesis is the
    A. type I hypothesis
    B. inferred hypothesis
    C. null hypothesis
    D. described hypothesis

43. The characteristic of research procedures that is demonstrated when a data collection instrument (such as a test) is given twice under the same circumstances and produces identical data is called
    A. validity
    B. reliability
    C. sensitivity
    D. appropriateness

44. If you want to make a month-to-month comparison of the number of coding errors by the coding staff, which of the following QI tools would provide an assessment of this raw data?
    A. cause-and-effect diagram
    B. flow chart
    C. histogram
    D. bar graph

45. The PDCA (Plan, Do, Check, Act) method was developed in the 1920s by _____.
    A. Brian Joiner
    B. Joseph Juran

C. W. Edwards Deming
D. Walter Shewhart

46. Referring to the chart of coding errors below, what would be the coding error rate for Wednesday for the total department?

Occurrences of Coding Errors

Coders	Mon	Tues	Wed	Thu	Fri	Weekly Total (individuals)
Madeline		1	1			2
Amanda	2		3	1		6
Emily		1		2	1	4
Daily Total	2	2	4	3	1	12

    A. .33%
    B. 33%
    C. 4%
    D. 40%

47. If you want to show how a process changes and fluctuates over a certain period of time, the CQI of choice would be a
    A. bar graph
    B. run chart
    C. pie chart
    D. pareto chart

48. This QI pioneer identified the 14 points for companies to follow for a successful quality improvement program
    A. Brian Joiner
    B. Joseph Juran
    C. W. Edwards Deming
    D. Walter Shewhart

49. You have noticed a problem with the filing of loose reports in the file area. As supervisor of the file area, you must find out the root causes for this problem. The QI tool that you should use would be the
    A. cause-and-effect diagram
    B. flow chart
    C. histogram
    D. bar graph

50. You are HIM director and need to give a report on the number of delinquent records coming into your department for the month of November. Which QI tool would be helpful in gathering this information?

    A. histogram

    B. decision matrix

    C. bar graph

    D. check sheet

51. The crude distance between scores is the

    A. interquartile range

    B. mode

    C. median

    D. range

52. Under PL 92-603, which information was not necessary to review by the UR/UM committee?

    A. Medicaid admissions

    B. Medicare admissions

    C. Blue Cross admissions

    D. Maternal and Child Health Program admissions

53. The kind of measurement scale that orders data into ranks is called

    A. nominal scale

    B. ordinal scale

    C. interval scale

    D. ratio scale

54. Merrytown Hospital's HIM department needs to investigate the number of incomplete records from January to June (6-month period), which will show if there are any patterns or trends for this time period. What QI tool is this?

    A. scatter diagram

    B. radar chart

    C. histogram

    D. run chart

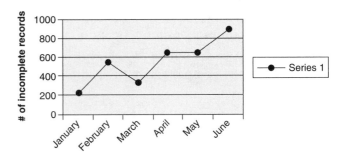

55. The cause-and-effect diagram is also known as the

    A. pareto chart

    B. scatter diagram

    C. fishbone diagram

    D. PDCA chart

56. You are HIM director and have noticed an increase in errors in your chart analysis clerks. After offering the chart analysis clerks an inservice, you would like to demonstrate that progress has been made and show before-and-after data. What QI tool would effectively display this before-and-after data and the progress made of these employees?

    A. scatter diagram

    B. radar chart

    C. histogram

    D. fishbone diagram

57. The terms "continuous quality improvement" and "quality assurance" are used interchangeably but are two different concepts. Which of the following would be characteristics of "continuous quality improvement?"

    A. emphasis is on monitoring whether the appropriate things are being done correctly with a focus on individual performance

    B. attention is first on the processes and causes

    C. the focus is on outliers, bad apples, and clinical outcomes

    D. all of the above

58. _____ was designed in 1997 to incorporate outcomes measurement and monitoring into the accreditation process for hospitals, long-term care organizations, and health care networks.
    A. JCAHO's ten-step process
    B. ORYX initiative
    C. National Committee for Quality Assurance
    D. Clinical Practice Guidelines

59. A(n) _____ is a measurement that targets events or patterns of events suggestive of a problematic process or behavior.
    A. threshold
    B. quality indicator
    C. performance measure
    D. variance

60. The QI pioneer who believed that training should be at top management to identify problems and opportunities for improvement, and then training of employees to assist in proposing and implementing solutions.
    A. Philip Crosby
    B. W. Edward Deming
    C. Brian Joiner
    D. Joseph Juran

61. Pareto charts
    A. display categories of data in descending order
    B. display how individual aspects relate to the whole
    C. display how often an event occurs
    D. display data over time

62. Which of the following represents the "Do" phase of the PDCA method?
    A. incorporate changes into department policies
    B. identify costs, people, and materials
    C. decide on improvement initiatives
    D. meet with staff to discuss changes

63. Your HIM department needs to chart trends in the response time to physician's record requests from the file clerks, which will compare patterns of occurrence over time. What QI tool is this?
    A. histogram
    B. pareto chart
    C. run chart
    D. scatter diagram

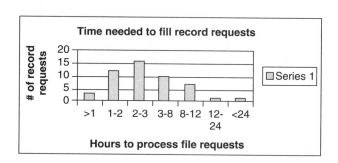

64. When you want to generate ideas on a particular subject and then incorporate a rating system for prioritizing ideas, you would use what QI tool?
    A. questionnaire/survey
    B. brainstorming
    C. Nominal Group Technique (NGT)
    D. check sheet

65. A tool used for achieving simultaneous goals of optimal care and appropriate resource utilization are called
    A. clinical pathways
    B. total quality management
    C. quality indicators
    D. clinical practice guidelines

66. The term used to mean the radical rethinking of the organization's processes rather than department performance is called
    A. redesigning
    B. change management
    C. reengineering
    D. none of the above

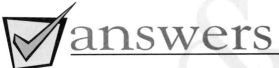

answers & rationales

1.

B. The two transcriptionists who work half time together make one FTE; therefore, there are five FTEs in the unit. Total productivity in the department is 5,150 lines per day. Dividing this total by the five FTEs gives the average production per day of 1,030 lines (Abdelhak, pp. 523–524).

2.

D. Although quality controls might be placed on the billing process from a management standpoint, billing is not strongly related to the quality of care provided to the patient (Abdelhak, pp. 374–375).

3.

D. While the plan would mention the fact that there is a utilization management coordinator (if, indeed, the hospital elected to have one), details such as the coordinator's responsibilities would usually not be included (Abdelhak, pp. 400–407; Johns, pp. 495–496).

4.

C. The risk management program may be a part of the hospitalwide quality management program. Continuing education programs for personnel are important in reducing risk (Abdelhak, pp. 408–410; Johns, p. 508).

5.

D. Although medical staff should participate in safety review, the review itself is a function of the hospi-tal (often through a Safety Committee) (Abdelhak, p. 384; Johns, p. 502).

6.

C. Answer A should only be a part of developing a frame of reference; answers B and D can also be very beneficial (Abdelhak, pp. 344–346).

7.

C. The review involves only studies that are similar to the proposed study. This literature can be very helpful in planning the research design (Abdelhak, p. 343).

8.

A. First, figure out how many workdays there are in 4 weeks if the unit is open Monday through Friday (5 days × 4 weeks = 20). Next, figure out how many lines must be transcribed, on average, per day (200,000 ÷ 20 = 10,000 lines). Finally, if the minimum standard per transcriptionist per day is 1,000, figure out how many transcriptionists are needed to type 10,000 lines per day (10,000 ÷ 1,000 = 10 FTEs) (Abdelhak, p. 523; Johns, pp. 735–736).

9.

A. PSROs were nonprofit professional licensed organizations composed of licensed physicians in an area. Their role has been assumed by QIOs (formerly PROs) arising out of the prospective payment system. JCAHO, formed in 1952, is a nongovernmental, nonprofit organization. The ACS (the American College of Surgeons) was founded in 1913 and carried the primary responsibility for hospital standardization until 1952, when JCAHO was organized (Johns, p. 255).

10.

B. Risk management seeks to prevent untoward events that cause certain malpractice actions as a response to the tremendous rise in insurance premiums for medical liability coverage that must be held by all hospitals. Risk management programs have had the added benefit of enhancing hospitals' quality management efforts (Abdelhak, pp. 407–412; Johns, pp. 500–511).

11.

A. Two types of criteria might be used: diagnosis/procedure-specific, or criteria related to severity of illness/intensity of service (the latter is used most often) (Abdelhak, p. 402; Johns, p. 495).

12.

A. The Medicare law (Title XVIII of the Social Security Act) was passed in 1965 (Abdelhak, p. 58; Johns, p. 495).

13.

D. See the Joiner Triangle in Cofer & Greeley's CQI for HIM (Cofer & Greeley, p. 20).

14.

B. The 10 steps are outlined in Abdelhak (p. 386).

15.

A. Risk management and quality management programs are not mandated by federal law. The Medicare law is PL 89–97 (Johns, pp. 255–266).

16.

B. Defining a service's major functions should be done before its important aspects of care are determined (Abdelhak, pp. 381–382).

17.

D. The hospital's plan might include provision for the other three (answers A, B, and C), but they were not required (Abdelhak, pp. 400–401; Johns, p. 497).

18.

A. Early resolution of incidents can prevent later court action (Abdelhak, pp. 410; Johns, pp. 502–503).

19.

C. Remember the generic rate used in health statistics: the number of times something did happen divided by the number of times it could have happened, times 100. In this case, the number of times something did happen (actual errors) is 156. The number of times it could have happened (there could have been errors in every line) is 2,586. Therefore, the rate is $156/2,856 \times 100 = 6.03\%$, considerably worse than the standard of 2% (Abdelhak, p. 309; Johns, p. 419).

20.

B. In return for a more stable and certain patient population, the hospital (or physician) reduces its (his or her) charges to the insurance plan. This agreement to reduce charges, in turn, encourages the hospital (or physician) to contain its (his or her) costs as effectively as possible. A member of a health maintenance organization can usually select from among a variety of providers (Abdelhak, pp. 43–44; Johns, p. 358).

21.

D. Accreditation, licensing, and certifying are all responsibilities of other organizations (e.g., JCAHO, state health departments, the American Osteopathic Association, etc.) (Abdelhak, pp. 248–249; Johns, pp. 271–272).

22.

A. The hazard surveillance checklist, usually completed by the hospital's safety officer or Safety

Committee, is used to identify potentially hazardous conditions (Abdelhak, p. 384).

23.

B. This project is entitled the Agenda for Change (Abdelhak, p. 376).

24.

A. Credentialing, or the granting of permission to provide patient care services, is based on several factors, including licensure, training, experience, and current competence (Abdelhak, pp. 465–466).

25.

B. Sometimes preadmission review or certification is limited to certain third-party payors and/or certain diagnoses or procedures (Abdelhak, p. 401).

26.

B. The physician reviewer may contact the attending physician to discuss the need for admission and to provide further documentation if necessary (Abdelhak, pp. 400–402).

27.

D. In contrast to incident reports, which identify institutional problems, occurrence screening identifies, concurrently or retrospectively, physician-related adverse patient occurrences (Abdelhak, pp. 410–411; Johns, p. 509).

28.

A. Even research that is not completed or results that do not agree with the hypothesis may still be of high quality. Both contribute to knowledge (Abdelhak, pp. 350–351).

29.

B. This is an example of underutilization (Abdelhak, pp. 400–407).

30.

B. The incident report facilitates the early identification of problems (Abdelhak, p. 410; Johns, pp. 502–503).

31.

A. Through the Medicare Conditions of Participation and through the activities of the Peer Review Organizations, Medicare has increasingly influenced quality management programs in hospitals (Abdelhak, pp. 413–415).

32.

D. Credentialing and blood usage review are examples of medical staff monitoring and evaluation. Dietetic review is an example of clinical service monitoring and evaluation (Abdelhak, p. 383).

33.

B. Exploratory studies seek to find ideas or insights. Often this approach serves as a preliminary study to help formulate the research hypothesis. Descriptive studies are intended to describe a certain set of conditions; no judgments are made. The testing of causal relationships is considered the most scientific of the three (Abdelhak, pp. 343–349).

34.

A. Comparative studies determine if there is a difference between two variables. Correlational designs determine the degree of difference between two variables (Abdelhak, pp. 398–399).

35.

C. Correlation is a data analysis technique. Observation involves watching a subject function in the research situation. Questioning involves posing questions to the subject, either by survey or by questionnaire. Measurement involves applying a device, such as a test or scale, to a subject (Abdelhak, pp. 398–399).

36.

B. Scatter diagrams are useful any time you want to see if a relationship exists between two variables (Cofer & Greeley, p. 87).

37.

D. Simple random sampling gives each member of a population an equal chance of being included. Stratified random sampling divides the population into two or more subpopulations, or strata. Cluster sampling applies simple or stratified methods repetitively until one arrives at the population elements that constitute the desired sample. Systematic sampling can be done when a complete list of all the elements in a population is known. The total number is divided by the desired sample size, and then the resulting answer is used to choose the sample systematically (Abdelhak, p. 338).

38.

A. A histogram is used to analyze trends or patterns over time (Abdelhak, p. 397; Cofer & Greeley, p. 65).

39.

C. Philip Crosby is a well-known quality consultant who established the "zero defects" philosophy (Abdelhak, p. 392; Cofer & Greeley, p. 19).

40.

C. The standard deviation measures the degree of variation in the same way, but is expressed in the same unit of measure as the original data (it is also the square root of the variance). The variance and the standard deviation are measures of dispersion and variability. The z-score is the standard score for comparisons across distributions; the t-score is the standard score in whole numbers. Both the z- and t-scores are measures of relative position (Abdelhak, pp. 328–329).

41.

D. A type II error occurs when a researcher fails to reject the null hypothesis when it is false (Abdelhak, p. 330).

42.

C. A null hypothesis is the reverse of what one expects to find, and states that there will be no differences between and among variables. If it can be shown that the null hypothesis is untrue (i.e., is rejected), the research hypothesis can be accepted with more confidence (Abdelhak, p. 330).

43.

B. Seven required characteristics of research procedure include reliability, validity, sensitivity, appropriateness, objectivity, feasibility, and ethical standards. These are difficult concepts, best explained in a research methods text (Abdelhak, pp. 340–355).

44.

D. Use a bar graph when you want to look at how different sets of data compare with each other. Cofer and Greeley's CQI Tools reference provides a diagram (p. 43; see also Abdelhak, p. 397).

45.

D. The PDCA method was developed by Walter Shewhart, who was an early QI pioneer. This tool is also referred to as the Deming Cycle (Abdelhak, p. 393; Cofer & Greeley, p. 74).

46.

B. To calculate the coding error rate for Wednesday, you divide 4 into 12 and multiply by 100 (Abdelhak, p. 249).

47.

B. A run chart displays the process of data over time (Abdelhak, p. 397; Cofer & Greeley, p. 82).

48.

C. W. Edwards Deming developed Deming's 14 points (Abdelhak, p. 391; Cofer & Greeley, p. 16).

49.

A. Cause-and-effect diagrams are useful for organizing and listing possible causes to identify root causes for a problem (Abdelhak, p. 396; Cofer & Greeley, p. 50).

50.

D. A check sheet is a grid that displays how often an event occurs (Cofer & Greeley, p. 54).

51.

D. The interquartile range is a measure of dispersion that represents the score that is at the 75th percentage minus that at the 25th percentage. It is used to adjust for instability in data. The range is also a measure of dispersion. The mode, median, and mean are all measures of central tendency (Abdelhak, pp. 325–328; Johns, pp. 423–426).

52.

C. Title XIX (Medicaid), Title XVIII (Medicare), and Title V (Maternal and Child Health Programs) patient admissions all had to be reviewed under PL 92–603 (Abdelhak, pp. 400–401; Johns, pp. 497–498).

53.

B. An example of an ordinal scale is Superior, Excellent, Good, Fair. A nominal scale uses named or labeled categories that are not ranked (e.g., Males, Females). An interval scale uses units with an equal interval between each unit (e.g., 30, 40, 50, 60). A ratio scale is like an interval scale but includes zero (e.g., $-10, -5, 0, 5, 10$) (Abdelhak, p. 322).

54.

D. A run chart is used when you want to look at trends over time and allows for quick assessment of performance trends and patterns. Like in this case, vacations or holidays can show variations in the number of record deficiencies due to doctor absences (Abdelhak, p. 397; Cofer & Greeley, p. 82).

55.

C. The cause-and-effect is also known as the fishbone diagram because the diagram looks like a fishbone. It was developed by Ishikawa (Abdelhak, p. 392; Cofer & Greeley, p. 50).

56.

B. A radar chart shows before-and-after data, which can show progress of the employees after the inservice (Cofer & Greeley, p. 80).

57.

B. According to Cofer and Greeley, "QA involves looking for problems retrospectively . . . CQI, on the other hand, involves ongoing proactive assessment and the reflection of error or imperfection at any level." Answers A and C are characteristics of the traditional QA approach (Abdelhak, p. 375; Cofer & Greeley, p. 15).

58.

B. ORYX was developed by JCAHO to be used as a continuous data collection tool for the accreditation process (Abdelhak, p. 386).

59.

B. The JCAHO defines an indicator as "a quantitative instrument that is used to measure the extent to which an organization or component thereof carries out the right processes, carries out those processes well, and achieves desired outcomes . . ." (Abdelhak, p. 386).

60.

C. Brian Joiner believed in training top management first and also developed the Joiner Triangle (Cofer & Greeley, p. 20).

61.

A. Answer A correctly describes pareto charts (Abdelhak, p. 397; Cofer & Greeley, p. 72).

62.

B. Identifying costs, people, and materials is part of the Do phase. Answer A is the Act phase. Answer C is the Plan phase. Answer D is the Check phase (Abdelhak, p. 393; Cofer & Greeley, p. 192).

63.

A. A histogram is a bar graph that can be helpful in analyzing trends and patterns of occurrence over time (Abdelhak, p. 397; Cofer & Greeley, p. 65).

64.

C. The Nominal Group Technique (NGT) uses brainstorming but takes it a step further by implementing a rating system for prioritizing a list of possible solutions (Abdelhak, p. 395; Cofer & Greeley, p. 70).

65.

A. Clinical pathways or care maps assist in providing standardized and routine delivery of patient care for the purpose of optimal and appropriate resource utilization. Quality indicators are events or patterns of events that are measured for variances. Clinical practice guidelines are statements to assist clinicians regarding appropriate patient care decisions (Abdelhak, pp. 386–388).

66.

C. Reengineering is the term used that has the same focus as continuous quality improvement and means "focused process improvement, major business process improvement and business process innovation . . ." rather than a departmental focus (Johns, p. 273).

10 Organization and Supervision

objectives

After completion of this chapter, the student will be able to:

➤ Explain the functions of supervision/management.

➤ Distinguish between the various types of plans utilized in supervision/management.

➤ Describe planning tools utilized in supervision/management.

➤ Explain the fundamentals of budgeting.

➤ Discuss ergonomics with regards to office space and environment planning in the HIM department.

➤ Explain the methods utilized to organize people.

➤ Identify techniques utilized for performance improvement.

➤ Utilize collection tools, data analysis, and data presentation techniques for performance and quality improvement in the HIM department.

DIRECTIONS (Questions 1–90): Each of the questions or incomplete statements below is followed by suggested answers or completions. Select the **best** answer in each case.

1. Before designing a new procedure to replace a current, inadequate one, the manager would NOT do which of the following?
   A. make a detailed analysis of the current procedure
   B. become thoroughly familiar with the current procedure
   C. discard the current procedure and write an entirely new one
   D. gather information about problems with the current procedure

2. One of the best sources for discovering problems with procedures is the
   A. medical staff
   B. department director
   C. director's immediate supervisor
   D. employees using the procedure

3. Which of the following would not be considered a scientific method of establishing standards?
   A. stopwatch studies
   B. work sampling
   C. personal experience
   D. time-log studies

4. The key consideration in planning the physical layout of a health information management department is
   A. productivity of employees
   B. work flow
   C. the budget
   D. lighting

5. A special tool that aids in the placement of equipment is the
   A. configuration chart
   B. office layout chart

   C. movement diagram
   D. flow process chart

6. Main aisles in an office should be at least
   A. 3 feet wide
   B. 5 feet wide
   C. 7 feet wide
   D. 8 feet wide

7. The concept indicating the limits placed on an individual's ability to decide on actions or to order actions from others is called
   A. delegation
   B. responsibility
   C. authority
   D. management

8. Which of the following would not cause delegation to fail?
   A. a sufficient amount of authority is not granted to the subordinate
   B. the subordinate is not held responsible for accomplishing the task
   C. the manager allows the subordinate to accept risk
   D. the manager does not define the results expected

9. The use of a good job description would not be useful information for which of the following?
   A. performance evaluation
   B. personnel selection
   C. preparing job orientation plans
   D. placement of equipment

10. An organization chart ensures good
    A. organization within the department
    B. management

C. visualization of the department's structure

D. line relationships

11. The first task in completing the work distribution chart is to

A. determine the job position of each employee

B. have each employee complete a list of his or her daily activities

C. have each supervisor complete a list of the daily activities of his or her subordinates

D. have the department director complete a list of the daily activities of each employee

12. The major advantage of effective controlling is that

A. employees are disciplined appropriately

B. plans are revised

C. activities are streamlined

D. problems are identified more quickly

13. A production monitor that is most disturbing to the employee is the

A. work flow chart

B. movement diagram

C. employee-reported log

D. stopwatch study

14. The first step in preparing a departmental budget is

A. counting the total number of hours the department will be open during the next fiscal period

B. reviewing the department's objectives for the next fiscal year

C. reviewing the supplies and equipment already on hand

D. determining how many hours employees will be on leave during the next fiscal period

15. Given the following information, compute the number of open shelving units needed. Each unit is 8 shelves high and 36 inches wide. The current file area houses 22,075 linear filing inches of records. The goal is to expand this by 10%.

A. 78 units

B. 85 units

C. 77 units

D. 84 units

16. Which of the following would not be normally factored in when preparing a budget?

A. a review of the effectiveness of the department's present operation

B. projections for growth in the facility's operations

C. changes in the patient turnover rate

D. a review of the qualifications of present employees

17. A health information management department with nearly full files wishes to purchase new shelving equipment. Currently it has 16,000 linear filing inches in use. It has been decided to add shelving that would provide an increase in filing inches of 25%. If each filing unit has 6 shelves of 33 inches per shelf, how many units should be purchased?

A. 21

B. 20

C. 202

D. 4,000

18. One way to encourage more productivity in a transcription unit is to

A. shorten the workday by an hour

B. vary the work assigned to each transcriptionist

C. place all transcriptionists on a part-time basis

D. have the desks of transcriptionists face each other

19. Which of the following is not included in the MBO cyclic process?
    A. organization
    B. feedback
    C. planning
    D. performance review

20. A supervisor over the assembly area in a health information management department has determined that one employee can assemble 15 charts per hour, on average. Assuming that an employee can work 1,850 hours per year (after allowing for vacation, holidays, etc.) and that there are 12,500 discharges expected during the next budget year, how many FTEs should the supervisor recommend the department have next year for the assembly function?
    A. 0.45
    B. 0.21
    C. 1.23
    D. 0.50

21. Depicting a chronological flow of work through graphic representation is done using a
    A. flow chart
    B. work sample
    C. work distribution chart
    D. PERT network

22. As a health information management department director, you are faced with the problem of a persistent backlog of work that you know is caused by a shortage of coding personnel. You've had several complaints from the business office about this problem. Your budget does not allow for overtime or for hiring additional personnel. Your own time is too limited for you to begin coding yourself. You do not wish to hurry your coders because their coding is of a reasonable speed and excellent quality. Which of the following

would NOT be considered a constraint in this problem that will affect your decision making?
    A. time
    B. money
    C. personalities
    D. quality

23. The hospital's revenue budget is usually prepared by the accounting department. The health information management department's contribution to revenue is usually limited to which of the following departmental functions?
    A. correspondence
    B. abstracting
    C. filing
    D. assembly

24. The crisis manager demonstrates poor ability in which management function?
    A. planning
    B. organizing
    C. controlling
    D. actuating

25. A type of budget that is created as if all activities of the organization or department were new is called a
    A. zero-based budget
    B. standard budget
    C. departmental budget
    D. zero-start budget

26. Which of the following is not included in a procedure document?
    A. title of the procedure
    B. effective date
    C. qualifications of the person performing the procedure
    D. statement giving the purpose of the task outlined in the procedure

27. All of the following signals could indicate a need to review a department's procedures EXCEPT:
    A. bottlenecks
    B. inadequate department forms
    C. new equipment
    D. lowered costs

28. One type of plan expressed in numerical terms is called a
    A. quantitative analysis
    B. budget
    C. quantitative procedure
    D. number policy

29. Health information management departments are usually organized according to the
    A. skills of the employees
    B. space configuration of the department
    C. functions performed
    D. accessibility to other departments

30. Positions that have direct responsibility for accomplishing the objectives of the organization are called
    A. line positions
    B. hierarchical positions
    C. direct-line positions
    D. staff positions

31. An organization chart may not be arranged according to
    A. job
    B. function
    C. either job or pay grade
    D. either job or function

32. The work distribution chart cannot show which of the following organizational problems?
    A. uneven distribution of benefits
    B. uneven distribution of work
    C. inappropriate specialization
    D. disproportionate use of time

33. The work distribution chart will show
    A. the exact way each moment of the day's time is spent by the employee
    B. the time spent by the employee within a 10% to 15% margin of discrepancy
    C. the best way to use equipment each day
    D. the exact way each moment of the day's time is spent by the employee, with the exception of recognized breaks

34. Which of the following is not an example of a control tool?
    A. work distribution charts
    B. performance standards
    C. variance analysis
    D. monitors

35. Counting the number of typographical errors in transcription is an example of what type of monitor?
    A. direct inspection
    B. work simplification
    C. work sampling
    D. quality control

36. During work sampling of a file clerk's activity, it is noted that out of 300 observations the employee is speaking on the telephone during 76 observations. How much of the employee's time is spent on the phone if the employee works 7 hours a day?
    A. 1.77 hours
    B. 3.28%
    C. 9.2%
    D. 3.94 hours

37. Budgets usually planned for the 12-month period are known as the
    A. calendar year
    B. functional year
    C. fiscal year
    D. accounting year

38. A health information management department director would NOT be expected to predict which of the following when preparing a budget?
   A. the number of personnel that will be required
   B. equipment needs
   C. the supplies that will be needed
   D. increases in Social Security taxes

39. The controlling power of the budget is exercised when a comparison is made between
   A. this year's projections and last year's projections
   B. next year's projections and last year's expenses
   C. this year's expenses and this year's budgeted expenses
   D. this year's budgeted expenses and next year's projections

40. Which solution given should be the last one used to solve a problem that becomes apparent from variance analysis?
   A. making adjustments in procedures
   B. redistributing workload
   C. hiring more staff
   D. providing more training

41. The source of power in which the follower perceives that the leader has special knowledge or expertise is called
   A. coercive power
   B. reward power
   C. referent power
   D. expert power

42. In a terminal digital filing system with 100,000 records, the goal is to have a file guide for every 50 records. How many guides should be purchased?
   A. 200
   B. 5,000

C. 500
D. 2,000

43. The hospital administrator requests a report on the number of cholecystectomies performed by a particular physician in April of the previous year. Of the following, the place to look for this information might be the
   A. patient register
   B. diagnostic index
   C. operating room register
   D. operation index

44. A health information management department director wishes to determine the usage of the health records being stored in an out-of-the-way area. Which of the following ratios would provide the information?
   A. $\dfrac{\text{Number of records filed}}{\text{Number of records stored}} \times 100$

   B. $\dfrac{\text{Number of requests received}}{\text{Number of records found}} \times 100$

   C. $\dfrac{\text{Number of records retrieved}}{\text{Number of records stored}}$

   D. $\dfrac{\text{Number of records retrieved}}{\text{Number of records stored}} \times 100$

45. As health information management department director, you wish to submit a capital budget request for five new open shelving units. The department's file area has enough space to hold the units. The present shelves are not adequate to hold records, and you do not wish to microfilm any closer to the current year. In preparing your request, your first task will be to describe
   A. the cost of the new shelves
   B. the need for the new shelves
   C. the shelving
   D. where the shelving will be placed

46. Leadership can be characterized as
   A. dominance given (through force or fear) to the leader by followers

B. a formal relationship of administrative control

C. dominance given (essentially voluntarily) to the leader by followers

D. manipulation of followers

47. Control methods that are combined with the planning process does not include which of the following?

A. PERT network

B. work distribution chart

C. budgets

D. MBO

48. File cabinets, desks, computer hardware, and typewriters are examples of

A. operational budget items

B. incremental budget items

C. capital budget items

D. supplies and expenses budget items

49. A small hospital's diagnosis and operation indexes currently include only the patient's number and the diagnosis and operation codes. The Utilization Management Committee would like to be able to use the indexes to help find records appropriate for their review. Which of the following data items should be added when records are abstracted for the indexes?

A. name of attending physician

B. date of admission

C. length of stay

D. age of the patient

50. A health information management department director notices that final autopsy protocols are not being sent to the department until 5 to 6 weeks after the autopsy was performed. He or she should

A. contact the Chief of Staff

B. consult with the hospital administrator

C. talk to the director of pathology

D. do nothing

51. Of the following, which is the step taken last in the problem analysis and decision-making process?

A. controlling the alternative solution chosen

B. gathering further information

C. defining how and when the alternative will be accomplished

D. choosing the solution to the problem

52. A department's operational plan is comprised of specific, verifiable

A. standards

B. procedures

C. objectives

D. rules

53. Departmental objectives should complement and supplement the

A. department director's professional goals

B. personal goals of the director's immediate supervisor

C. hospital's goals

D. goals of other departments in the hospital

54. In the policy, "If possible, no more than two employees of the health information management department should be on vacation at one time," which phrase encourages the use of the manager's judgment?

A. health information management department

B. vacation

C. employees

D. if possible

55. In procedure writing, the steps in the procedure should be

A. as detailed as possible

B. sequenced with the easiest steps to perform at the beginning

C. kept to a minimum

D. arranged with those steps taking the most time sequenced first

56. Which of the following is false about procedures?
    A. reviewed against actual performance periodically
    B. assigned to only one employee at a time
    C. designed to ensure uniformity of practice
    D. they should be specific to a task

57. A planning technique in which the flow of planning moves from the bottom of the organizational hierarchy up is called
    A. goal-oriented management
    B. objective-oriented management
    C. management by objectives
    D. democratic management

58. Effective work flow means that
    A. employees are provided an appropriate amount of work
    B. paperwork moves in as straight a line as possible
    C. productivity is measured in units of work accomplished per hour
    D. employees are provided with an adequate supply of materials to perform the work

59. When planning an office, which of the following should not be considered?
    A. a supervisor should be placed at the back of the employees he or she supervises
    B. employees' desks should be placed so that employees face each other, if possible
    C. the file area should not be placed near the department entrance
    D. employees dealing with people outside the department should be placed near the department's entrance

60. A disadvantage of informal organization include which of the following?
    A. communication may be enhanced
    B. a safety valve for employee frustrations is developed
    C. social values of the informal organization may work against the formal organization's objectives
    D. employees' personal satisfaction may be increased

61. Possible errors in organization that an organization chart cannot point out are which of the following?
    A. spans of control that are too large
    B. duplication of functions
    C. lines of authority that overlap
    D. spans of control that contain unequal numbers of employees

62. Meeting objectives through the cooperation of employees is the major objective of which function of management?
    A. planning
    B. organizing
    C. controlling
    D. directing

63. An approach to determining leadership style that plots concern for people against concern for production is the
    A. hierarchy of needs
    B. flow process chart
    C. managerial grid
    D. two-factor diagram

64. It is suggested that a specific time of day be set, after which routine requisitions for health records to be pulled for the following day will not be accepted. One factor that might determine what time of day should be set (noon or 4:00 p.m., for example) is
    A. the size of the file area
    B. the number of charts being requested
    C. the person requesting the charts
    D. scheduling of file room personnel

65. Certain records are better filed in an area where health information management

department personnel other than the director cannot have access to them. Which of the following would not be included?

A. psychiatric records

B. records of health information management department personnel

C. records of famous persons

D. records involving legal actions against the facility or members of the medical staff

66. Which of the following would not be considered a constraint that may impede planning on the part of the health information management department director?

A. his or her superior's attitude toward change

B. provision in the next budget for an additional employee

C. interdepartmental relationships

D. medical staff

67. In designing a microfilm system, which of the following should be considered last?

A. the type of equipment to be used for storage of the microfilm

B. the nature of the information being microfilmed

C. how large the documents to be filmed are

D. how the microfilm can best be organized

68. Budgeting for depreciable equipment is part of

A. operational budgeting

B. capital budgeting

C. zero-based budgeting

D. incremental budgeting

69. A transcription supervisor has received permission to expand her unit by one extra person. She has a small but steady backlog of discharge summaries. Her transcriptionists, all excellent employees, handle all of the functions of the unit, including preparing reports for transport to the units, mailing, etc.

The supervisor also does some transcription when her time is not exhausted by supervisory duties. She should hire

A. another full-time transcriptionist

B. an assistant supervisor

C. a transcriptionist who specializes in discharge summaries

D. a clerk-typist

70. Which of the following tasks could NOT be delegated by a coding supervisor to an experienced coder?

A. preparing a weekly productivity report for the department director

B. ordering supplies

C. performance appraisal

D. serving on a departmental quality improvement team

71. In problem analysis and decision making, asking an employee to note how often he or she answers the telephone each day is an example of which task?

A. proposing alternative solutions to the problem

B. gathering relevant data

C. choosing the best alternative

D. making the decision

72. A strategic plan would be used for

A. developing and/or revising the mission statement

B. developing next year's budget

C. developing a new smoking policy

D. developing a new release of information policy

73. An effective policy requires which of the following by the manager?

A. judgment

B. strict adherence

C. diversification

D. manipulation

74. Procedures provide for
    A. flexibility in performing a task
    B. guidelines for designing a policy
    C. standardization in performing a task
    D. interpretation while performing a task

75. One reason for collecting procedures into a procedure manual might be
    A. to satisfy state law
    B. to aid in cross-training of employees
    C. to keep procedures from getting lost
    D. to allow easy review by the medical staff

76. One way to initiate or manage change in the workplace is (are) through
    A. job redesign
    B. job enlargement
    C. job enrichment
    D. job descriptions

77. Work simplification is mainly a part of which function of management?
    A. planning
    B. organizing
    C. leading
    D. controlling

78. Which of the following is not a step in goal setting as an operational planning technique?
    A. the setting of objectives by subordinates
    B. setting the goals
    C. providing support (e.g., equipment, time, etc.)
    D. obtaining commitment to the goals

79. Employees' desks should be
    A. 5 to 6 feet apart
    B. 1 to 2 feet apart
    C. 0 to 2 feet apart
    D. 2.5 to 3 feet apart

80. Positions of responsibility that involve assisting and advising others are called
    A. line positions
    B. advisory positions
    C. consultant positions
    D. staff positions

81. Authority developed by an employee that is NOT delegated is called
    A. assumed authority
    B. informal authority
    C. attained authority
    D. token authority

82. A department's organization chart cannot show employees which of the following?
    A. the quality of management in the department
    B. possible lines of promotion
    C. their organizational relationship to other employees
    D. the limits of their authority and responsibility

83. Which is not considered (in addition to the statute of limitations) in determining when a health record may be destroyed?
    A. the readmission rate
    B. costs involved in microfilming, inactive storage, and destruction
    C. the volume of research done in the facility
    D. the number of physicians on the medical staff

84. Given the following members of a health information management department, who would find color coding of health record folders most helpful?
    A. director
    B. filing room supervisor
    C. quality assurance coordinator
    D. coding supervisor

85. A coder notices that an attending physician's progress notes do not indicate the fact that the patient's temperature was rising and that the white count was abnormal. When the matter is brought to the physician's attention by the health information management department director, the physician states that the notes are satisfactory. The matter should now be
    A. dropped altogether
    B. referred to the Quality Management Committee
    C. referred to the Chief of Staff
    D. referred to the Health Record/HIM Committee

86. A transcriptionist's line count per day has dropped significantly over the past 2 weeks, causing a backlog in histories and physicals and several angry phone calls from physicians and the operating room supervisor. The transcription supervisor should
    A. fire the transcriptionist
    B. refer the matter to the director of the health information management department (the supervisor's superior)
    C. speak to the transcriptionist privately
    D. suspend the transcriptionist for a few days

87. As a filing room supervisor, you employ a file clerk who is about 55 years old, has worked in the file room for many years, but has gradually become dissatisfied. This employee is not interested in further education or in learning a new job. Ways in which you might be able to help the employee include all of the following EXCEPT:
    A. delegation of special assignments
    B. consulting the employee on various problems
    C. constructive criticism
    D. asking the employee to teach others

88. The director of nursing services decides that the file clerks in the health information management department must share weekend coverage in order to relieve the weekend supervisory nurses of the task of finding records. This decision is
    A. reasonable, given the director's authority
    B. inappropriate
    C. responsible, given the supervisory demands of the weekend nurses
    D. fair if the file clerks want extra work

89. A filing supervisor wishes to find out how well records are being found in the file area. A ratio to be used could be
    A. $\dfrac{\text{Number of records not found}}{\text{Number of records requested}} \times 100$
    B. $\dfrac{\text{Number of records filed}}{\text{Number of records not found}} \times 100$
    C. $\dfrac{\text{Number of records filed}}{\text{Number of records found}} \times 100$
    D. $\dfrac{\text{Number of records found}}{\text{Number of records not found}} \times 100$

90. As director of the health information management department, you manage the department through four supervisors who collectively supervise all of the functions of the department. One day you notice a senior coder quickly code a health record from the face sheet and then turn to the next record, code again from the face sheet, and turn to a third record. You should
    A. do nothing
    B. carefully discuss the problem with the coder, pointing out the error and explaining the value of the correct procedure
    C. discuss the problem with your supervisor because of its implications for reimbursement
    D. discuss the problem with the coder's supervisor

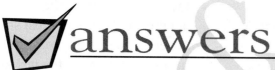

answers & rationales

1.

C. Often parts of the older procedure can be retained (Abdelhak, p. 549).

2.

D. Employees using the procedure will be able to identify possible problems and can offer solutions for improvement (Abdelhak, pp. 549–550).

3.

C. Personal experience is likely to be more subjective than the other three, which rely on objective measurement of job performance (Abdelhak pp. 524–526).

4.

B. Proper layout can help add to productivity by increasing efficiency and attractiveness. The major factor in planning, however, is the way work flows through the department (Abdelhak pp. 550, 553–554; Johns, p. 721).

5.

A. A configuration chart can be especially useful when there are many pieces of interrelated equipment placed in physically separate areas, such as a multi-user computer system (Abdelhak, pp. 544–548).

6.

B. Secondary aisles should be at least 3 feet wide (Abdelhak, p. 557).

7.

C. Employees should have a clear indication of how much authority they have (Abdelhak, p. 492; Johns, pp. 731, 742).

8.

C. Allowing the subordinate to make mistakes is necessary to successful delegation (Abdelhak, pp. 492–494; Johns, pp. 731, 742).

9.

D. Placement of equipment is better done through a physical layout. Good job descriptions can also facilitate the investigation of employee grievances and the determination of appropriate pay (Abdelhak, pp. 502–512; Johns, pp. 734–735, 740).

10.

C. The organization chart helps to visualize the structure of the departments within an organization or good line relationships but does not ensure that they exist (Abdelhak, p. 540; Johns, pp. 718–721).

11.

B. Since the employee is the person best able to keep track of his or her activity, each employee should make a personal daily activity list (Abdelhak, pp. 518–523).

12.

D. Answers A, B, and C are possible consequences of follow-up activities associated with the controlling function, but they are not advantages of the function itself. During the controlling phase, activities are measured. Problems can be identified if and when they arise (Abdelhak, pp. 502–506).

13.

D. The stopwatch study can be distorted both by the employee (who either artificially paces his or her work or becomes so nervous that the results are inaccurate) and by the supervisor (who can appear intimidating in this role) (Abdelhak, pp. 524–526).

14.

B. Once objectives are reviewed, a determination of what resources will be needed to accomplish the objectives must be made: employees and the hours they work; equipment and supplies, both on hand and to be acquired; etc. (Abdelhak, p. 542).

15.

B. Each open shelving unit holds $8 \times 36 = 288$ linear filing inches of records. A 10% expansion of current filing inches equals $22,075 \times 0.10 = 2,207.5$ extra inches. Then $22,075 + 2,207.5 = 24,282.5$ inches needed altogether to allow for the 10% expansion. The next step is to divide the total inches needed by the inches in one shelving unit: $24,282.5 \div 288 = 84.31$ units. This answer must be raised to the next whole number, 85 units (Abdelhak, p. 182; Johns, p. 788).

16.

D. While a change in the qualifications of present employees might be expected to alter a budget (e.g., a clerk-typist, on passing the accreditation exam, might be promoted and given a salary increase), present qualifications will not alter next year's budget. Patient turnover rate reflects the rapidity with which patients are admitted to the facility (Abdelhak, pp. 630–631).

17.

A. First, figure out how many additional linear filing inches will be needed ($25\% \times 16,000 = 4,000$).

Then determine how many filing inches are in each unit (6 shelves $\times$ 33 inches per shelf = 198) and divide the inches needed (4,000) by the inches per unit ($4,000 \div 198 = 20.2$). The answer must be increased to 21 units in order to accommodate the entire 4,000 inches (Abdelhak, pp. 557; Johns, p. 790).

18.

B. Varying the work by combining different types of reports, different lengths of reports, different dictators, and different levels of difficulty within a transcriptionist's workload will help reduce monotony (Abdelhak, pp. 526–527; Johns, pp. 521, 523).

19.

A. In the planning phase, goals and objectives are defined: some by the manager, some by the subordinate, and still others by both. In the performance review phase, both manager and subordinate evaluate the progress toward goals and objectives or modify them as necessary. In the feedback phase, the manager reviews overall organizational and departmental goals for the next planning period, as well as initiating corrective action (Abdelhak, pp. 599, 605).

20.

A. The formula would be: 12,500 discharges per year divided by (15 charts per hour $\times$ 1,850 hours) = 0.45 FTEs (Abdelhak, p. 523).

21.

A. The flow chart can be used for planning procedures and activities in detail, or it can be used as a controlling tool to compare actual work flow with the original plan (Abdelhak, p. 531).

22.

C. You are constrained by time (the business office needs the codes being held up; you lack time for coding), money (budgetary restraints on overtime or more personnel), and quality (which you do not want to sacrifice for speed). There is nothing in the problem to suggest a personality constraint (complaints from the business office are not due to their personalities, but to your problem) (Abdelhak, p. 505).

23.

A. Revenue refers to the income of the organization. Health information management departments bring in revenue directly as a result of the search and copying charges resulting from answering requests for release of information (the correspondence function) (Abdelhak, p. 637).

24.

A. The crisis manager has not thought ahead to plan for potential problems (Bernstein, p. 1).

25.

A. In a zero-based budget, each activity must be justified anew (Abdelhak, p. 630; Johns, p. 751).

26.

C. Qualifications required to fill positions are included in job descriptions. The procedure should also list the tools or materials required to perform the task (with attached samples, if possible) and the procedural steps themselves (Abdelhak, pp. 590–591).

27.

D. Lowered costs usually indicate improvement in productivity, efficiency, and/or effectiveness; they are sometimes a result of procedure revision (Abdelhak, p. 542).

28.

B. A budget is also a control (Abdelhak, p. 628; Johns, p. 796).

29.

C. Because employees change far more often than functions, organizing a department according to the skills of particular employees creates frequent problems (Abdelhak, pp. 531, 534).

30.

A. They are termed line positions because together they form a hierarchy within an organization, with each position reporting to a level above (Johns, pp. 718–719).

31.

C. Although often a chart will fall into an order such that higher-paid employees are closer to the top of the chart than lower-paid employees, this is due to the authority, skill, or training required by a function rather than a deliberate arrangement (Abdelhak, p. 540; Johns, p. 718).

32.

A. Work distribution charts do not correlate compensation (wages and benefits) with amount or type of work (Abdelhak, p. 518).

33.

B. The chart would become too complex if every interruption were included. In addition, the chart does not make allowances for fatigue or for delays due to factors outside the employee's control (e.g., a mainframe computer system may have several users at once, thus slowing its response time) (Abdelhak, pp. 518–523).

34.

A. Work distribution charts do not measure an employee's quality of work or efficiency (Abdelhak, pp. 518–523).

35.

A. Monitors are a component of quality control. Work sampling is a production monitor rather than a quality monitor, and might instead be used to measure the quantity of transcription produced. (Abdelhak, p. 524–526; Johns, pp. 521–523).

36.

A. The percentage of time spent equals (76 divided by 300) × 100 = 25.3%; 25.3% of 7 hours = 7 × 0.253 = 1.77 hours (Abdelhak, pp. 524–526; Johns, pp. 521–523).

37.

C. The fiscal year can run from January to December (the calendar year) or for any 12-month period. Another common fiscal year is July 1 through June 30 (Abdelhak, p. 640).

38.

D. Tax costs are usually added organizationally rather than departmentally (Abdelhak, p. 630; Johns, p. 796).

39.

C. The comparison of what is usually spent and what was budgeted to be spent as a result of various predictions and projections is one way the department's performance can be evaluated (Abdelhak, p. 487).

40.

C. Hiring more staff is costly and may not be necessary; the other solutions should be considered first (Abdelhak, pp. 630–631; Johns, p. 796).

41.

D. Much of a health information management practitioner's power derives from this source (Abdelhak, p. 492).

42.

D. The answer is determined by dividing the number of records (100,000) by 50 to arrive at 2,000 guides. The type of filing system is not an issue in this question (Abdelhak, pp. 182–184; Johns, pp. 787–788).

43.

D. The operation index lists all of the cholecystectomies done during the month in question. Computerized indexes almost always indicate the physician in each case, so that finding a particular surgeon's cases is not difficult. Most manual systems also indicate the surgeon (Johns, pp. 140, 206).

44.

D. Answer C is incorrect, since a ratio implies a percentage, and therefore the answer obtained from the division calculation must be multiplied by 100. An example might be: 60 records were retrieved from the storage area in a one-month period. There are approximately 20,000 records stored in the area. The ratio would be (60 × 100) ÷ 20,000 = 0.3%. Answer A is incorrect, since records filed might include new records as well as records being refiled after use. The number of requests received (answer B) would not necessarily equal the number of records pulled, because requested records might not be in the storage area, but already signed out of the hospital for microfilming, etc. (Abdelhak, p. 182; Johns, p. 788).

45.

B. A description of your realistic assessment of the need for the shelves will help the governing body prioritize your request among the many others it receives (Abdelhak, pp. 627–631; Johns, p. 796).

46.

C. Answers A and D are implied in the concept of power. Answer B is a characteristic of authority. Leadership is the act of influencing individuals to meet objectives (Abdelhak, p. 499; Johns, pp. 727, 732).

47.

B. Work distribution charts involve an evaluation of the organization. Gantt charts also combine controlling and planning (Abdelhak, p. 518).

48.

C. Capital items are those that are usually over $500 to $1,000 in cost (the actual figure is determined by each organization) and that last for several years.

Operational budgets comprise a supply and expense budget and a personnel budget (Abdelhak, pp. 644–645).

49.

C. Because one of the UM Committee's concerns is the lengths of stay of patients relative to their diagnoses, including the length of stay will help the committee choose records that are unusual in this respect (Abdelhak, pp. 402–407; Johns, pp. 495–497).

50.

D. The complete, final autopsy report or protocol should be in the health record within 60 days (about 8 1/2 weeks). A preliminary report of provisional and anatomic diagnoses should be recorded within 72 hours and placed in the record (Abdelhak, p. 95).

51.

A. Follow-up (a type of control) is necessary to evaluate whether the objective is being accomplished (Johns, pp. 731–732).

52.

C. Objectives and goals are sometimes used interchangeably; some authors refer to objectives as more specific than, and derived from, goals (Abdelhak, p. 487; Johns, pp. 729–730).

53.

C. The goals of all departments and the medical staff should reflect their basis in the hospital's mission and goals (Abdelhak, p. 486).

54.

D. The inclusion of the phrase "if possible" gives the manager the opportunity to allow more than two employees to take vacation at the same time if he or she believes that the circumstances warrant the exception to the policy (Johns, pp. 736, 792–795).

55.

C. The number of steps should be kept to the minimum necessary for carrying out the procedure. Too much detail makes procedures far too long. The sequence of the procedure should be chronological. If this allows some flexibility in arrangement (e.g., the order of certain steps does not matter), then steps that are similar should be grouped together (Abdelhak, p. 549; Johns, p. 736–737).

56.

B. Several employees may use the same procedure at one time (Abdelhak, p. 549; Johns, pp. 736–737).

57.

C. Management by objectives (MBO) can be effective in allowing everyone to participate in defining the organization's future, thereby increasing commitment to the organization's objectives. MBO is also considered a control technique (i.e., performance appraisal) and can be used with individual employees in the department as well (Abdelhak, p. 488).

58.

B. Paperwork should also move as short a distance as possible at one time. Answer C is one definition of a standard that would apply to certain functions (e.g., charts assembled per hour, lines transcribed per hour) (Abdelhak, p. 536).

59.

B. This arrangement encourages talking and provides many other distractions to employees (Abdelhak, pp. 550–554).

60.

C. This might occur when individuals not holding the same social values as the informal group feel like outcasts or when the informal group's social values lead to resistance to change (Abdelhak, pp. 540–541).

61.

D. Spans of control may appropriately be of different sizes due to the nature of the work done. The or-

ganization chart can also show inefficient alloca-
tion of personnel and a lack of intermediate supervisory levels (Abdelhak, p. 540; Johns, p. 718).

62.

D. Directing is also called actuating, ordering, and several other terms (Abdelhak, p. 499; Johns, p. 732).

63.

C. The managerial grid is useful in classifying various managerial styles, but it does not help in
determining the cause behind a particular classification (McDonnell-Brown, p. 1).

64.

D. If file room personnel are scheduled to work in the
evenings, for example, then requests for records to
be ready for the following morning can still be handled even if the requests are received late in the af-
ternoon. If the file area is not staffed in the evening,
however, the records will have to be pulled in the af-
ternoon, so a deadline of noon would be more appropriate (Johns, pp. 787–788).

65.

A. A locked file cabinet in the director's office is a
common storage place for sensitive records (Huffman, p. 303).

66.

B. The clue in this question is the word *may*. Answers
A, C, and D may impede planning, or they may not.
However, a new employee can only enhance planning, since a new employee can contribute to many
plans the director might like to implement (Abdelhak, pp. 485–488; Johns, p. 726).

67.

A. Until answers B through D and several others (such
as money available to operate the system, where
the microfilm will be housed, etc.) are known, the
type of storage equipment cannot be appropriately
determined (Abdelhak, p. 209).

68.

B. The capital budget includes items and projects that
are costly, last for a long time (usually over 1 year),
and can be depreciated (Abdelhak, pp. 644–645;
Johns, p. 796).

69.

D. The clue to this answer lies in the fact that highly
trained transcriptionists are performing the cleri-
cal functions of preparing reports for transport to
the nursing units and for mailing. The supervisor
could better schedule this work with a clerk-
typist, freeing up time for the transcriptionists to
clear up the backlog. Because her employees are
excellent, more supervision in the form of an assistant supervisor is probably unnecessary
(Abdelhak, pp. 518–526).

70.

C. Supervisory functions that involve the authority
to approve, recommend, or implement matters relating to employees should be retained by the supervisor. All of these tasks are part of the
performance appraisal process. It would be unfair
and inappropriate for an employee to appraise the
performance of other employees on the same organizational level. A productivity report (answer
A) is merely a factual compilation of data; interpretation of the data and its reflection on the performance of the coders would be the function of
the supervisor (Abdelhak, pp. 492–494; Johns,
pp. 731, 742).

71.

B. This information might also be needed to define
the problem further (perhaps the employee is a
coder who appears to be frequently interrupted by
the telephone). Answers C and D are essentially the
same thing (Johns, pp. 731–732).

72.

A. Answer B would use a financial plan; answers C
and D would use an operational plan (Abdelhak,
p. 487; Johns, p. 727).

73.

A. Policies are broad guidelines; they require some interpretation, depending on the circumstances surrounding the decision that must be made (Abdelhak, p. 548).

74.

C. Procedures help standardize tasks so that different persons performing the same task perform it in the same way. Unlike policies, procedures allow little flexibility or interpretation; they are more rigid than policies and serve as guides to action only (Abdelhak, p. 549; Johns, p. 718).

75.

B. Having the department's procedures collected together provides a useful reference to the tasks performed by the department. Although policy and procedure manuals are probably not of interest to the medical staff, surveyors from licensing and accrediting agencies might ask to see them (Abdelhak, pp. 548–549; Johns, pp. 792–795).

76.

A. Change management is the term used for supervisors implementing change in the workplace. Job redesign is a tool to use to initiate change (Johns, p. 748).

77.

C. Leading involves getting all members of the work group to contribute to the achievement of organizational objectives in the most effective and efficient way. Work simplification is a scientific approach to leading (Abdelhak, p. 499; Johns, p. 743).

78.

A. Answer A is a feature of management by objectives (MBO) (Abdelhak, p. 488).

79.

D. Desks placed too closely together facilitate unnecessary conversation and can cause noise problems (e.g., when one employee is using the telephone or is typing). Desks placed too far apart can result in poor utilization of space (Abdelhak, pp. 554–557).

80.

D. Staff positions might include those in marketing, personnel, or planning (Abdelhak, p. 540).

81.

B. Informal authority is often the result of an employee's seniority, intelligence, or skill at interpersonal relationships. This authority can be helpful to the manager in getting changes accepted by department employees (Abdelhak, p. 492).

82.

A. Quality of performance (management, productivity, interpersonal skills, etc.) cannot be demonstrated on an organization chart (Abdelhak, pp. 178–179).

83.

D. If patients (inpatients and outpatients) tend to be readmitted quite often, records should be retained for a longer period. The greater the amount of research being done in a facility, the longer the retention period should be (Abdelhak, pp. 183–184; Johns, pp. 786–788).

84.

B. Color coding helps to prevent misfiles in the filing of health records. Of the four department members given, the filing room supervisor would find color coding the most helpful in checking the quality of filing being done (Abdelhak, pp. 183–185; Johns, pp. 786–788).

85.

D. The Health Record/HIM Committee is responsible for analyzing and evaluating the quality of the health record. Although the Health Record/HIM Committee might wish to pursue the matter further, to include the Quality Management Committee, the

Chief of Staff, or others, this problem in documentation should be referred to the Health Record/HIM Committee (if there is one in the hospital) by the health information management department director (Abdelhak, p. 104).

86.

C. Why is the transcriptionist's productivity lessening? Despite the serious consequences of her lack of productivity (e.g., the backlog of histories and physicals and the angry responses from others), the supervisor should consider the possibility of problems that might be affecting the transcriptionist's productivity before taking any of the more serious measures given in the other answers (Abdelhak, pp. 524–526).

87.

C. The employee has not done anything wrong, so criticism of any sort is inappropriate. This individual has been sometimes called a dead-end employee, one who can go no further in the organization and who has exhausted the material rewards that might help motivate. Using the long experience of this type of employee as a basis for providing extra status and prestige to the employee may help with motivation (Abdelhak, pp. 607–610; Johns, p. 745).

88.

B. The decision is inappropriate (even if it might be a good idea), because the director has exceeded her authority by making decisions about employees not under her supervision. She should forward her idea to the health information management department director and let that individual act on it in an appropriate way (Abdelhak, pp. 607–610; Johns, p. 745).

89.

A. For example, if 10 times during the past month a record was not found out of the 1,000 that were requested, the ratio would be 10 (1000 × 100 = 1%). The generic formula for any ratio is: the number of times something did happen divided by the number of times something could have happened, multiplied by 100. In this case, the number of times charts were not found (something did happen) was divided by the number of charts requested (theoretically, it would have been possible for *all* of the requested charts to be not found) (Abdelhak, pp. 183–184; Johns, pp. 786–788).

90.

D. The manager should not jump the chain of command by correcting a problem with an employee not directly subordinate to him or her. Doing so violates the principle of unity of command and undermines the authority delegated to the supervisor. There are exceptions to this situation, however, particularly if there is a safety issue involved and quick corrective action is required (Abdelhak, pp. 489–490).

11 Human Resources

objectives

After completion of this chapter, the student will be able to:

➤ Describe job descriptions, job enlargement, and job enrichment.

➤ Identify recruitment techniques in human resources management.

➤ Discuss the interview process and appropriate practices.

➤ Describe labor relations with regards to union activities.

➤ Describe the federal labor laws.

➤ Discuss wage and salary administration.

➤ Explain performance appraisals.

➤ Describe the disciplinary action steps.

DIRECTIONS (Questions 1–87): Each of the questions or incomplete statements below is followed by suggested answers or completions. Select the **best** answer in each case.

1. If a standard in a health information management department is that a coder on average can code 27 records per day, and the hospital discharges, on average, 72 charts per day, how many FTE coders does the department need?
   A. 2.7
   B. 0.4
   C. 3.0
   D. 2.0

2. Which is not a motivating technique?
   A. money
   B. behavior modification
   C. quality circles
   D. problem solving

3. Which is not included in compensation?
   A. fringe benefits
   B. salary
   C. incentives
   D. equipment

4. A scheduling technique that allows a full-time position to be shared among two or more employees is called (a)
   A. flextime
   B. job sharing
   C. multipart job
   D. multi-employee job

5. If an employee has a serious personal problem that is interfering with his or her work performance, the supervisor might refer the employee to the
   A. OSHA
   B. FLSA
   C. NLRB
   D. EAP

6. The theory of motivation that suggests that every action is motivated by an unsatisfied need is called
   A. theory X and theory Y
   B. the two-factor theory
   C. the hierarchy of needs
   D. the incentive theory

7. A barrier to effective communication might be
   A. a lack of common meaning in the language used
   B. a common frame of reference
   C. too few organizational levels through which information must flow
   D. feedback

8. The Fair Labor Standards Act is the
   A. federal Wage and Hour law
   B. law that allowed bargaining units in not-for-profit hospitals
   C. law that modified the Social Security Act
   D. law that set up cafeteria-style benefits packages

9. Which of the following does not significantly affect the span of control?
   A. complexity of the work
   B. physical location of the work units
   C. manager's level within the organizational hierarchy
   D. unity of command

10. Modifying the content of a job so that an employee has a wider variety of tasks, increased responsibility, and greater opportunity for recognition is called
    A. job content analysis
    B. job control
    C. job enrichment
    D. methods improvement

11. Departmental orientation should not include which of the following?
    A. the role and function of the department in the hospital
    B. hospital fire prevention rules
    C. departmental policies and rules
    D. departmental organization

12. Another term for *negative discipline* is
    A. written warning
    B. oral reprimand
    C. punishment
    D. criticism

13. If an employee approaches his or her supervisor with what the employee considers a grievance, the supervisor should listen to the employee and then
    A. ignore it if it is only a minor complaint
    B. put the complaint aside to see if other employees complain about the same thing
    C. deal with the complaint only if the employee seldom complains
    D. deal with the complaint as a bona fide grievance

14. Which is not an external resource?
    A. money
    B. machinery
    C. labor
    D. motivation

15. The process of finding easier and better ways to perform work is called
    A. flow process
    B. work simplification
    C. work distribution
    D. work flow

16. Which of the following is not included in a job description?
    A. the tools or materials the position holder needs
    B. the title of the job or position
    C. the qualifications of the position
    D. the effective date

17. A criterion against which performance can be measured is characteristic of
    A. schedules
    B. procedures
    C. job descriptions
    D. standards

18. The number of employees who can be supervised effectively by one person is not dependent on which of the following?
    A. the amount of subordinate training
    B. the nature of the work being supervised
    C. the age of the employees being supervised
    D. the necessity for frequent communication

19. An advantage of informal organization includes which of the following?
    A. members of the informal group may be afforded status
    B. communication among the informal group may undermine morale
    C. frustrations expressed within the informal group may become self-fulfilling
    D. informal groups may become resistant to change

20. Job enrichment means that
    A. the employee is given more opportunities for decision making and participation without more work
    B. the employee is given more jobs to vary the work and make it less dull and routine
    C. employees meet voluntarily and regularly to solve work problems
    D. specific goals are set, regular feedback is provided, and recognition and praise are awarded

21. When evaluating an employee's performance, the supervisor should
    A. point out the employee's strengths
    B. restrict his or her comments to areas that need improvement
    C. assume that the employee has done only the minimum necessary to obtain a satisfactory evaluation
    D. share the evaluation with the employee only when there might be a problem with the employee's performance

22. Training an employee to perform tasks usually done by another is called
    A. counter-training
    B. cooperative training
    C. cross-training
    D. retraining

23. When the salary structure is based on actual work produced, the pay system is called a (an)
    A. productive pay system
    B. wage pay system
    C. utilization pay system
    D. incentive pay system

24. A manager who believes that employees inherently dislike work; must be persuaded, rewarded, or punished in order to modify their behavior; and want to avoid responsibility subscribes to
    A. theory X
    B. theory Y
    C. two-factor theory
    D. hierarchy of needs

25. Which of the following is a required fringe benefit?
    A. relocation expenses
    B. medical insurance
    C. overtime pay for nonexempt employees
    D. pension plans

26. In wage and salary administration, the determination of the relative value of each job in the facility is called job
    A. description
    B. analysis
    C. control
    D. evaluation

27. Which of the following are not indications that training of employees might be needed?
    A. new equipment
    B. changes in policies
    C. new services
    D. improved quality of work

28. The federal agency that regulates employee safety and health issues is
    A. OSHA
    B. NLRB
    C. EEOC
    D. SSA

29. As HIM Director, you are faced with a problem employee and must take disiciplinary action. What would the usual first step in applying discipline for a first offense be?
    A. termination
    B. suspension
    C. oral reprimand
    D. written warning

30. The most important task in handling grievances is
    A. making a quick decision
    B. writing down a description of the grievance
    C. getting information about the grievance
    D. notifying the personnel department director about the grievance

31. The requirement for unemployment compensation was established with the
    A. Fair Labor Standards Act
    B. Social Security Act

C. Civil Rights Act

D. Occupational Health and Safety Act

32. The laws that prohibit discrimination in employment because of race, color, religion, sex, or national origin are called

A. fair labor standards laws

B. equal pay laws

C. equal employment opportunity laws

D. rehabilitation laws

33. During a union organizing campaign, the supervisor can do which of the following?

A. question prospective employees about past union affiliations

B. tell employees about the disadvantages of belonging to a union

C. attempt to prevent internal organizers from soliciting memberships during non-working time

D. discriminate against prounion employees

34. External resources include which of the following?

A. creativity

B. equipment

C. perseverance

D. negotiation skills

35. A flow process chart is used to

A. determine how long an employee spends on a task

B. outline each step within a task

C. show how equipment is placed

D. show the materials used in performing a task

36. The need for improvement in a procedure would NOT show up graphically on the flow process chart by which of the following?

A. frequent delays

B. excessive transportation

C. repetitious inspections

D. individuals who are too highly qualified performing certain steps

37. Rules should apply to

A. employees on probation

B. nonsupervisory personnel

C. nonadministrative personnel

D. all personnel

38. A process that determines the content of a job is called

A. writing a job description

B. job analysis

C. procedure analysis

D. work simplification

39. The document that shows how much time employees spend on various activities is called a (an)

A. organization chart

B. flow chart

C. work process chart

D. work distribution chart

40. Which one of the following questions CANNOT be answered by analysis of a work distribution chart?

A. Is a task disproportionately divided among employees?

B. Is time being spent on unnecessary tasks?

C. Are the skills of each employee being utilized appropriately?

D. Are employees reporting to the most appropriate supervisor in terms of the supervisor's expertise?

41. A process based on probability theory, whereby work is spot-checked, is called

A. work simplification

B. work distribution

C. flow process

D. work sampling

42. An organization's statement of philosophy is a (an)
    A. organizational concept
    B. plan
    C. measure of assessment of progress toward a goal or objective
    D. standard

43. Work simplification cannot be achieved by which of the following?
    A. reducing the distances traveled by people or paper
    B. combining work activities where possible
    C. reducing employee involvement in the process
    D. eliminating unnecessary steps in the process

44. Which of the following questions may NOT be asked at an interview with an applicant for a job?
    A. Which responsibility in your last job gave you the most trouble?
    B. I see that you were in the army. Did you receive an honorable discharge?
    C. Why did you leave your last position?
    D. When would you be available to begin work?

45. The true objective of discipline is
    A. punishment designed to prevent recurrence of the inappropriate behavior
    B. correction of the inappropriate behavior
    C. to reinforce the relationship between superior and subordinate
    D. to avoid favoritism on the part of the superior

46. The greatest resource a health information management department director has is
    A. adequate space
    B. employees
    C. computers
    D. a cooperative medical staff

47. Methods improvement could be used effectively when
    A. procedures have not been reviewed in the past year
    B. poor morale is evident
    C. costs are lower than expected
    D. no nonproductive activities are associated with the job

48. Employers may NOT pay unequal pay for equal work performed under similar working conditions because of which of the following?
    A. merit of the employee
    B. seniority of the employee
    C. sex of the employee
    D. incentive compensation system

49. During a union organizing campaign, the supervisor cannot
    A. ask employees about organizing activities or union matters
    B. insist that all organizing be done outside of working time
    C. inform employees that the institution can legally hire a replacement for an employee who strikes for economic reasons
    D. let employees know that signing a union authorization card is not a commitment to vote for the union if there is an election

50. When criticizing an employee, the focus should be on the employee's
    A. attitude
    B. behavior
    C. personality
    D. character

51. Methods of personnel selection may not include which of the following?
    A. application form
    B. candidate experience
    C. age of the candidate
    D. references

52. The impetus behind any disciplinary action should be
    A. to remove undesirable employees
    B. to prevent undesirable behavior from spreading among employees
    C. to punish the employee
    D. to change undesirable behavior in the employee being disciplined

53. An exempt employee is not paid
    A. incentive pay
    B. bonus pay
    C. overtime pay
    D. benefits

54. Which of the following does NOT have to be offered to employees?
    A. unemployment compensation
    B. life insurance
    C. worker's compensation
    D. Social Security

55. Grievances CANNOT be reduced by which of the following?
    A. supervisory and management personnel following established policies and procedures
    B. supervisory and management personnel keeping their promises
    C. employees understanding that their complaints will receive prompt attention
    D. employees understanding that only major problems should be forwarded to supervisory and management personnel

56. Which of the following problems would NOT best be resolved through the use of a group, task force, or committee?
    A. determining the best answer to a coding question
    B. determining the cause of delays in getting health records to the health information

management department from the nursing units after discharge
    C. whether a new form should be allowed to be used in the health record
    D. deciding on a new physician delinquency or suspension policy

57. Employers are required to make an extra effort to hire and promote individuals considered to be in a protected class (e.g., Native Americans, African Americans, women). This is called
    A. affirmative action
    B. minority hiring rule
    C. equal opportunity
    D. civil rights

58. Qualifications required to hold a particular position, as given in the job description, should be
    A. the maximum qualifications necessary
    B. the maximum qualifications that the position's supervisor would like the position holder to have
    C. the minimum qualifications needed to perform the job
    D. the minimum qualifications needed for promotion from that position to another

59. An HIM manager might determine standards in all of the following ways EXCEPT:
    A. simulation
    B. scientific or quantitative methods
    C. consulting the medical staff
    D. past performance records

60. A useful display technique that assists in designing work flow is a
    A. flow process chart
    B. work sampling observation record
    C. work distribution chart
    D. movement diagram

61. The concept that an employee is responsible to only one supervisor is called
    A. span of control
    B. unity of responsibility
    C. unity of command
    D. chain of command

62. The right of the employees to expect support from their superiors is part of the concept of
    A. authority
    B. span of control
    C. unity of command
    D. informal organization

63. The work distribution chart can show a need for review and possible revision of
    A. policies
    B. rules
    C. procedures
    D. lines of authority

64. When developing a work distribution chart, the supervisor should explain to subordinates that this is NOT an attempt to check on the
    A. employee's workload
    B. tasks the employee performs
    C. employee's productivity
    D. time spent on each task

65. In Maslow's hierarchy of needs, the highest level of need is for
    A. safety
    B. self-actualization
    C. esteem
    D. acceptance

66. Job enlargement means
    A. the employee is given more opportunities for decision making and participation
    B. the employee is given more jobs to vary the work and make it less dull and routine
    C. employees meet voluntarily and regularly to solve work problems

    D. specific goals are set, regular feedback is provided, and recognition and praise are awarded

67. Which of the following is not a factor in determining compensation?
    A. budgetary constraints
    B. managerial level of the employee's supervisor
    C. availability of people with the required qualifications
    D. pay scales of competitors

68. In work sampling, the selection of the times during which observation is to be made should be done
    A. sequentially
    B. randomly
    C. periodically
    D. continuously

69. Before criticizing an employee, the supervisor should first
    A. consult with his or her superior
    B. put everything in writing
    C. ask how he or she might have contributed to the problem
    D. wait until other employees can be asked about the situation

70. The Fair Labor Standards Act considers which of the following types of employees exempt?
    A. professional
    B. hourly
    C. executive
    D. administrative

71. During a union organizing campaign, the supervisor CANNOT
    A. give employees his or her opinions about unions
    B. keep outside organizers off the institution's premises

C. attend union meetings

D. tell employees about the disadvantages of belonging to a union

72. During a union organizing campaign, the supervisor can do which of the following?

   A. question employees about whether they have or have not signed a union authorization card

   B. give employees uncomplimentary factual information about the union or its officials

   C. grant pay raises to keep the union out

   D. visit the employees at home to urge them to oppose the union

73. Counseling interviews should be

   A. conducted with more than one supervisory person present

   B. documented

   C. judgmental

   D. conducted by human resources personnel

74. One prerequisite for job enrichment is that

   A. the supervisor must be experienced in job enrichment before attempting it on his or her own

   B. the supervisor's own job must be enriched before he or she can enrich employees' jobs

   C. the employees must want to participate

   D. the supervisor must be willing to delegate this responsibility to one of the employees in his or her span of control

75. Usual sources of applicants for job openings in hospitals would NOT include which of the following?

   A. television advertisements

   B. newspaper and journal advertisements

   C. employment agencies

   D. employee referrals

76. Approaches to job evaluation would NOT include which of the following?

   A. point system

   B. job ranking method

C. job classification method

D. ordering

77. During an interview with an applicant, the supervisor should NOT avoid which of the following?

   A. talking down to or above an applicant

   B. asking questions that encourage a "yes" or "no" answer

   C. interrupting occasionally

   D. phrasing questions so that an expected answer is encouraged

78. The objectives of an effective departmental orientation program does NOT include assisting the new employee to do which of the following?

   A. feel at ease with the department, new job, and new associates

   B. understand the function of the department and the role of his or her job in fulfilling that function

   C. understand the politics and personalities of his or her new associates

   D. understand the rules and regulations of the department

79. If oral or written warnings have not succeeded in altering inappropriate behavior, the final step before termination of the employee is

   A. reprimand by the director of the personnel department

   B. reprimand by the hospital administrator

   C. suspension

   D. demotion

80. The number of employees who report to a supervisor is called the

   A. span of control

   B. element of control

   C. supervisory effective number

   D. unity of command

81. Which of the following solutions uses the most resources?
    A. hiring extra staff
    B. updating procedures
    C. improving methods
    D. redistributing work

82. A program in which transcriptionists, for example, are rewarded for productivity of acceptable quality that exceeds established quantitative standards is called a (an)
    A. incentive program
    B. plus program
    C. fair productivity program
    D. control program

83. The visual tool that compares the relationship of work planned, work completed, and time is a
    A. work distribution chart
    B. flow process chart
    C. PERT network
    D. Gantt chart

84. A planning, coordinating, and controlling tool used with large, complex tasks that are nonrepetitive and require integration of several projects is called a
    A. flow process chart
    B. flow chart
    C. PERT network
    D. work sample

85. A form of fact gathering based on many observations made at random during a period of time is called
    A. work distribution
    B. work sampling
    C. random work choice
    D. interval work distribution

86. When giving an oral warning (or counseling), the supervisor should not do which of the following?
    A. provide exact details of the problem
    B. give the employee a chance to answer the charge
    C. place written notes about the incident in the employee's file in the personnel department
    D. acknowledge the positive aspects of the employee's behavior

87. Which of the following could not be analyzed using work sampling?
    A. determining the downtime of a machine
    B. determining the percentage of an employee's time spent on each activity
    C. determining the sequence of activities in an employee's task
    D. determining patterns of interference in the work flow

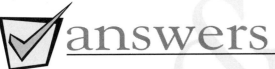

answers & rationales

1.

A. 72 charts per day ÷ 27 charts per coder = 2.67 or 2.7 FTEs. Although employees as individuals must be represented by whole numbers (i.e., answer C), FTEs can be measured in partial numbers. For example, two full-time coders, one part-time coder who worked only 0.5 or one-half of the usual full-time hours, and another part-time coder who worked 0.2 or one-fifth of the usual full-time hours, equal 2.7 FTEs but 4 individual employees. See Abdelhak, p. 254, for a formula.

2.

D. Problem solving may result from appropriate use of the other three (and other) techniques (Abdelhak, pp. 496–499; Johns, pp. 731–732).

3.

D. Compensation involves the financially related benefits of working as an employee of an organization. Equipment, although necessary for performing a job, still belongs to the organization (Abdelhak, pp. 611–612).

4.

B. Flextime allows employees to control their own work schedules within certain parameters (e.g., that the employee must be present between 10:00 A.M. and 2:30 P.M.). Answers C and D are fabricated (Abdelhak, p. 567).

5.

D. EAPs, or Employee Assistant Programs, are organized departments (usually part of Human Resources) staffed by social workers and other professionals that assist employees with personal issues in a confidential environment. OSHA (Occupational Safety and Health Administration) is the federal agency that ensures compliance with occupational safety and health regulations. The FLSA (Fair Labor Standards Act) requires a minimum wage (determined by Congress) and overtime compensation. The NLRB (National Labor Relations Board) adjudicates unfair labor practices (Abdelhak, pp. 572, 578–580, 583–584, 608).

6.

C. Maslow's hierarchy of needs states that once a need is satisfied, another level of need must be appealed to in order to motivate workers. The hierarchy begins with lower-order physiological needs, safety needs, and belonging needs, and proceeds to the higher-order needs of status and self-actualization. Answer D is a fabrication. Health information administration students should review Herzberg's two-factor theory and McGregor's theory X and theory Y (Norwood, p. 1).

7.

A. The other three enhance effective communication. Answer C is related to the fact that the fewer times a message must be relayed, the more effective the communication (Johns, p. 531).

8.

A. The FLSA sets a minimum wage (actually decided by Congress) and overtime pay regulations (Abdelhak, p. 572).

9.

D. The more complex the work is, the smaller the span should be. If units under the supervision of one individual are physically separated, the span should be narrower. The higher the manager's level within the organization's hierarchy, the more complex the work, thus the span should be smaller. The unity of command is a different principle, related to the desirability of having a subordinate report to only one superior (Abdelhak, pp. 490–491).

10.

C. Methods improvement may improve one task within a job or may make the job more efficient, but it does not have the motivational potential of job enrichment. The idea behind job enrichment is that the source of motivation is the job itself (2000 Accel-Team.Com, p. 1).

11.

B. This is better done at a hospitalwide orientation meeting when the hospital's safety officer is available to provide orientation. The new employee should also be oriented to the location of various facilities (locker room, restrooms) and to the general job functions he or she will be performing (Abdelhak, p. 598).

12.

C. Punishment may be the least effective way to discipline an employee, the object of which is to correct the inappropriate behavior (Abdelhak, pp. 607–610; Johns, p. 745).

13.

D. Bona fide grievances against an employer, outlined in a union contract or in the facility's personnel policies, should be handled according to hospital policy. Other complaints, even if the supervisor recognizes that they are not in the same category as a major grievance, should still be considered carefully (Abdelhak, pp. 608, 610–611; Johns, p. 746).

14.

D. Motivation is an internal resource (Stuarte-Kotze, p. 1).

15.

B. A flow process chart, better work distribution, and improved work flow may all contribute to work simplification (Abdelhak, pp. 526–527).

16.

A. These are given in procedures. The job description should also include who the person reports to, a summary of the position, and a list of routine tasks that make up the job. Other items (hours, salary, working conditions, line of promotion) can also be included (Abdelhak, pp. 506–512).

17.

D. Standards are important in planning schedules and determining staffing needs (Abdelhak, pp. 524–526; Johns, pp. 735–736).

18.

C. The span is less if the employees being supervised are performing different functions and/or difficult or detailed work (Abdelhak, pp. 490–491).

19.

A. This status may provide a sense of belonging and may contribute to personal satisfaction (Abdelhak, pp. 724–726).

20.

A. Job enrichment makes work more challenging and meaningful. Answer B is a description of job enlargement (2000 Accel-Team.Com, p. 1).

21.

A. Employees need praise as well as corrective guidance. All performance evaluations should be shared with the employee, who is naturally interested in how the supervisor perceives his or her performance (Abdelhak, p. 599).

22.

C. Cross-training is a form of in-service (Abdelhak, p. 586).

23.

D. Considerations involved in the implementation of incentive pay plans are discussed in Abdelhak (pp. 523–526).

24.

A. McGregor's theory Y manager, however, believes that employees do not inherently dislike work, that employees have a capacity for assuming responsibility, and that employees want to satisfy social, esteem, and self-actualization needs (NetMBA, p. 1).

25.

C. Overtime pay is required for nonexempt employees (Abdelhak, p. 572).

26.

D. Job evaluation is an equitable method of measuring the financial worth of jobs (Abdelhak, p. 612).

27.

D. Any major change can initiate the need for training. Answer D is one desired result of training (Abdelhak, pp. 615–617; Johns, p. 747).

28.

A. The Occupational Safety and Health Administration establishes standards, conducts workplace inspections, and imposes penalties as required by law (Abdelhak, p. 9; Johns, p. 506).

29.

C. The supervisor, through use of the oral reprimand or warning, seeks to stop the inappropriate behav-

ior at the start before it is repeated. The supervisor should provide complete privacy, a well-planned agenda, enough time, and a positive attitude. Flagrant offenses such as theft or fighting are dealt with more severely, often by firing the employee (termination of employment) (Abdelhak, pp. 607–610; Johns, p. 745).

30.

C. Thorough information is necessary before making a decision, because even a decision about even a minor matter may set a precedent (Abdelhak, pp. 610–611; Johns, p. 746).

31.

B. Individual states operate their own unemployment compensation plans, which vary significantly (West's Encyclopedia of Law, p. 1).

32.

C. Abdelhak lists these laws on p. 572 (see also, Johns, p. 507).

33.

B. These disadvantages might be strikes, picket-line duty, dues, fines and assessments, rule by a single person or small group, and possible domination of a local by its international union. Discrimination (answer D) can be involved in granting pay increases, apportioning overtime, making work assignments, promotions, layoffs, or demotions, or in the application of disciplinary action (Abdelhak, p. 581).

34.

B. Answers A, C, and D are managerial traits resulting from personality, character, experience, and education. They are intangible. Equipment is an external resource (Reh, p. 1).

35.

B. Answer A is determined by a work distribution chart, answer C by either a physical layout or a configuration chart, and answer D by a written procedure (Abdelhak, pp. 528–529; Johns, pp. 736–737).

36.

D. This might be remarked on in passing but will not be illustrated graphically. This information is better discovered from a comparison of the procedure with relevant job descriptions (Abdelhak, pp. 528–529; Johns, pp. 736–737).

37.

D. In a hospital, rules should also be followed by medical staff, volunteers, and visitors (Huffman, p. 665).

38.

B. A job description is the written result of job analysis (Abdelhak, p. 590; Johns, p. 734).

39.

D. This chart can be used, along with the organization chart, to review departmental organization (Abdelhak, pp. 518–523).

40.

D. The work distribution chart does not show organizational relationships or their quality. This question would have to be answered through analysis of the organization chart and relevant job descriptions and resumes. Other questions that the work distribution chart can answer are: (1) Is the work evenly distributed? (2) Is the time spent on various tasks reasonable and in line with their importance? (3) Are employees performing too many unrelated tasks? (Abdelhak, pp. 518–523).

41.

D. The key to accurate work sampling is in selecting the number of observations made and how they are made (Abdelhak, p. 524).

42.

B. Answers C and D can be the same thing and are concepts of control. The statement of philosophy (mission statement, creed, pledge, etc.) is a statement of the common values of the individuals who make up an organization and the purpose of the organization that is derived from those values. It is the most idealistic and abstract of all plans (Abdelhak, pp. 480–481; Johns, pp. 721–723).

43.

C. Effective efforts to simplify work activities require the willing participation of employees involved, as well as their knowledge of the work activities to be simplified (Abdelhak, pp. 526–527).

44.

B. Questions about skills or experience acquired while in the service are acceptable; questions about whether discharge was honorable, dishonorable, general, etc., are not (Abdelhak, pp. 595–597; Johns, pp. 738–739).

45.

B. Disciplinary action (e.g., written warnings) should outline how the employee can correct the problem. Avoiding favoritism (answer D) is an important guideline to ensure fair discipline, but it is not the goal or reason behind discipline (Abdelhak, pp. 607–610; Johns, p. 745).

46.

B. Without good employees, motivated and performing reasonably well, none of the other resources can be utilized (Abdelhak, p. 476).

47.

B. Methods improvement is another term for work simplification. Poor morale can result, for example, from a method that is too dependent on another's untimely input. Procedures that have not been reviewed can still have adequate methods. Answers C and D generally do not require improvement (Abdelhak, pp. 526–527).

48.

C. The other factors must be established as bona fide systems, and the inequality must be directly attributable to the system of merit, seniority, or an incentive plan (Abdelhak, p. 576).

49.

A. Employees may volunteer this information, and the supervisor may listen, but he or she cannot ask (Abdelhak, p. 581).

50.

B. Attitude, personality, and/or character may be impossible to change, but inappropriate behaviors can be corrected (Abdelhak, pp. 610–611; Johns, p. 746).

51.

C. Age, date of birth, sex, race, religion, and national origin are some of the criteria that cannot be used as means of selecting among candidates (Abdelhak, pp. 593–597; Johns, pp. 738–740).

52.

D. Answer B might be a secondary benefit of discipline in that employees will see that inappropriate behavior will result in disciplinary action, but the major reason for resorting to discipline should always be to try to change undesirable or inappropriate behavior (Abdelhak, pp. 610–611; Johns, p. 746).

53.

C. Exempt positions as classified by the Fair Labor Standards Act include executive, administrative, and professional positions (Abdelhak, p. 577).

54.

B. Life insurance is a fringe benefit that an organization may or may not offer (Symmetry Software Corp., p. 1).

55.

D. If employees understand that all grievances will be attended to, rather than only major ones, the supervisor will receive better communication about minor problems before they become major and far more difficult to handle (Abdelhak, pp. 610–611; Johns, pp. 745–746).

56.

A. This problem is best addressed by one or two people in the health information management department. The others are all too complex to be resolved without the interaction or recommendations of several people, including those outside the health information management department (Johns, p. 741).

57.

A. Affirmative action seeks to encourage both hiring and promotion of members of groups that have been discriminated against in the past in hiring and promotion decisions. The term is used only in the employment of individuals. Equal opportunity includes opportunities in education, housing, etc. (Abdelhak, p. 573).

58.

C. Recommended higher qualifications may be given, but the minimum qualifications allow preliminary screening of job applicants without difficulty and with more efficiency (Abdelhak, p. 506).

59.

C. Other ways include appraisal (or, more accurately, guessing) and review of literature (Abdelhak, p. 524; Johns, pp. 735–736).

60.

D. The movement diagram is usually superimposed on an office layout and illustrates motion through space (movement of paperwork through the office) (Abdelhak, p. 531).

61.

C. Contradictory orders and buck passing can result if more than one person is allowed to supervise a particular employee (Abdelhak, pp. 489–490).

62.

A. Authority works both ways, giving the employee the right to carry out assigned duties and to expect support when those duties are carried out within the employee's scope of authority (Abdelhak, p. 492).

63.

C. It can also point out problems in job descriptions (e.g., the qualifications for the work performed in a job may not be appropriate for the tasks comprising the job) (Abdelhak, pp. 518–523).

64.

C. Work distribution charts do not measure an employee's quality of work or efficiency (Abdelhak, pp. 518–523).

65.

B. The hierarchy moves from physiological needs (hunger, thirst) through security or safety, to acceptance, esteem or status, and self-actualization (Norwood, p. 2).

66.

B. Job enlargement can have negative results if the employee does not desire it. Answer A characterizes job enrichment. Answer C is a feature of quality improvement teams. Answer D lists features of behavior modification (Accel-Team.Com, p. 1)

67.

B. The Fair Labor Standards Act also influences compensation, as does performance of the employee (Abdelhak, pp. 611–615).

68.

B. Because work sampling is based on the statistical principle that observations made at random will provide just as complete information as continuous observations, a random sample of observations, based on the selection of random times at which an observation is made, should be the basis of the study (Abdelhak, p. 524).

69.

C. Problems requiring criticism may be partly due to poor training, poor actuating, poor response to communication, etc., all problems contributed to by the supervisor. Although writing the incident down (answer B) may be beneficial, this should be done both before and after criticism is made. Criticism is the business of the supervisor and the employee, not other employees. The supervisor should not rely on hearsay when considering criticism, but only on what he or she perceives with his or her own senses (answer D) (Abdelhak, pp. 607–610; Johns, p. 745).

70.

B. Exempt employees do not receive overtime pay (Abdelhak, p. 577).

71.

C. The supervisor also cannot participate in any undercover activities in order to find out who is or is not participating in union activities (Abdelhak, p. 581).

72.

B. The supervisor can also express his or her opinions on unions, union policies, or union leaders (Abdelhak, p. 581).

73.

B. Initial documentation might be restricted to the supervisor's file, while repeated or more serious problems might require placing documentation in the employee's personnel file (Abdelhak, pp. 610–611; Johns, p. 745).

74.

C. If employees are resistant to the idea of job enrichment, the effort will probably fail (Accel-Team.Com, p. 1).

75.

A. Television advertisements are prohibitively expensive. Other sources include the front door (walk-in applicants), write-in applicants, promotions and transfers, supervisors and department heads, job fairs, etc. (Abdelhak, pp. 592–593).

76.

D. The point system, in which certain factors (education, experience, responsibility, working conditions, etc.) are given numerical point values and used as a basis for evaluating jobs as sums of their points, is the most common. Salary grade is assigned according to the total point value of the job. In the job classification method, a predetermined number of job classes are established, and jobs are assigned to these classifications. In job ranking, jobs are arranged according to their difficulty. A fourth method of job evaluation is factor comparison (Abdelhak, pp. 612–615).

77.

C. If the applicant strays away from the question or rambles for a long time, the interviewer should interrupt in order to redirect the applicant's comments. Answer D is a definition of asking leading questions (Abdelhak, pp. 595–597).

78.

C. Discussion of employees' characteristics, personalities, friendships, cliques, etc., is inappropriate in a formal orientation program. The employee should be allowed to discover these with as little formal input as possible, although much will be absorbed informally from other employees (Abdelhak, p. 598).

79.

C. The supervisor with authority to discipline via oral or written warnings should also have the authority to suspend or fire the employee. Consulting his or her superior or the personnel or human resources director is appropriate and probably desirable, but the supervisor should administer the discipline (Abdelhak, pp. 610–612; Johns, p. 745).

80.

A. Span of control is also called span of authority or span of management. Unity of command refers to the theory of reporting to one boss. Answers B and C are not management terms (Abdelhak, pp. 489–491).

81.

A. Often, adding major resources such as employees or equipment isn't needed, while performing the other three activities might solve the problem using resources already available (Abdelhak, p. 651).

82.

A. An incentive (often monetary, or perhaps extra time off, a written commendation, or public acknowledgment) is offered as a reward for exceptional service (Abdelhak, pp. 599–605).

83.

D. The amount of time a certain activity should require is estimated and is plotted on the chart. Entries are added to the chart as work is completed. The chart shows how much has been done and how much remains to be done in order to meet the goal. The chart can be arranged to follow production in an area, individual employee production, or the productivity of a machine. Work distribution charts and flow process charts do not emphasize the planning relationships of activity versus time (Abdelhak, pp. 542–546).

84.

C. Abdelhak illustrates a PERT network for installing a new dictation system. The PERT network charts the plan and progress of this type of complex project (Abdelhak, pp. 542–546).

85.

B. The technique consists of periodic, frequent spot checks of employees, a piece of equipment, or an activity. The observations are recorded and then analyzed (Abdelhak, p. 524).

86.

C. Although the supervisor should document the incident and the meeting with the employee, these should be kept in the employee's file in the department at this point. A copy of a formal written warning is usually forwarded to the personnel (human resources) department (Abdelhak, p. 609).

87.

C. This would be done with a flow process chart, which follows each step in an activity sequentially. Work sampling only samples activities at discrete points in time (Abdelhak, p. 524).

12 Biomedical Sciences

objectives

After completion of this chapter, the student will be able to:

➤ Discuss the structure and function of the human body.

➤ Explain the pathophysiology of diseases.

➤ Describe diagnostic and treatment modalities and pharmacy therapy available in patient care management.

DIRECTIONS (Questions 1–76): Each of the questions or incomplete statements below is followed by suggested answers or completions. Select the **best** answer in each case.

1. The absence of blood supply to tissues is a condition known as
   A. caseation
   B. anoxia
   C. infarct
   D. necrosis

2. Which of the following groups of organs has the greatest role in maintaining homeostasis in the body?
   A. kidney, lung, liver
   B. liver, heart, intestine
   C. lung, liver, heart
   D. heart, kidney, intestine

3. Observation of the occurrence of disease in populations is
   A. epidemiology
   B. pathology
   C. sociopathology
   D. demography

4. Fat-soluble vitamins include
   A. A, D, E, and K
   B. B, C, and K
   C. A, C, and E
   D. C, E, and K

5. In idiopathic disease, the cause is
   A. an environmental factor
   B. a virus
   C. unknown
   D. systemic

6. The complaints of the patient, either voluntary or elicited by questioning, are referred to as
   A. signs
   B. lesions
   C. symptoms
   D. physical findings

7. When lymphatic or venous drainage in the leg is partially blocked, a result is
   A. dehydration
   B. edema
   C. effusion
   D. ascites

8. Occlusion of part of the cardiovascular system by impaction of a foreign mass transported to the site through the bloodstream is a (an)
   A. thrombus
   B. varicosity
   C. infarction
   D. embolism

9. When there is interference with the exchange of gases in the pulmonary alveoli, with an insufficient amount of carbon dioxide leaving the body, the result is
   A. respiratory alkalosis
   B. respiratory failure
   C. respiratory acidosis
   D. pneumonia

10. All of the following are causes of shock EXCEPT:
    A. loss of blood volume
    B. vasodilation
    C. sepsis
    D. first-degree burn

11. Scarlet fever is caused by a
    A. streptococcus
    B. staphylococcus

C. gram-negative bacillus

D. virus

12. Caseation, cavity formation, fibrosis, and calcification are the progressive stages of
   A. tuberculosis
   B. leprosy
   C. syphilis
   D. rheumatic fever

13. The presence of a chancre indicates the presence of which bacteria?
   A. *Bacillus pyocyaneus*
   B. *Mycobacterium leprae*
   C. *Treponema pallidum*
   D. *Escherichia coli*

14. The fungal infection causing thrush is
   A. mucosis
   B. dermatomycosis
   C. histoplasmosis
   D. *Candida*

15. The greatest public health problem in the world is caused by the
   A. trematodes
   B. *Plasmodium malariae*
   C. trypanosomes
   D. Pediculi

16. In healing by first intention the
   A. cut margins of a wound are brought together
   B. wound is treated with warm soaks
   C. cut margins are not brought together
   D. wound is left open to the air

17. Two types of cells important in the immune response are
   A. antigens and lymphocytes
   B. lymphocytes and cells of the reticuloendothelial system

C. T cells and lymphocytes

D. B cells and lymphocytes

18. An increase in the response to a particular antigen that is more severe than a normal reaction is called
   A. hypersensitivity
   B. hyperallergy
   C. hyperproductivity reaction
   D. excessive antibody reaction

19. Coumadin would be prescribed if the patient has what diagnosis?
   A. deep vein thrombosis
   B. gastroesophageal reflux
   C. cirrhosis
   D. congestive heart failure

20. The cause of death in cholera is mainly
   A. excessive vomiting
   B. hemorrhage
   C. dehydration
   D. peritonitis

21. Ringworm is a
   A. blastomycosis
   B. dermatomycosis
   C. mycoringosis
   D. cryptococcosis

22. All of the following are malignant tumors EXCEPT:
   A. sarcoma
   B. carcinoma
   C. glioma
   D. angioma

23. Two types of anaerobic bacterial diseases are
   A. tuberculosis and leprosy
   B. diphtheria and gonorrhea
   C. tetanus and gas gangrene
   D. botulism and typhoid fever

24. A disease acquired from infected animals, particularly cattle and goats, is
    A. erysipelas
    B. brucellosis
    C. Legionnaire's disease
    D. rheumatic fever

25. All of the following groups include only viral diseases EXCEPT:
    A. poliomyelitis, hepatitis A, rabies, yellow fever
    B. rubella, mumps, herpes simplex, varicella
    C. shingles, smallpox, mononucleosis, influenza
    D. encephalitis, rubeola, hepatitis B, tetanus

26. A malignant tumor that may reproduce the normal arrangement of cells is said to be
    A. differentiated
    B. anaplastic
    C. sarcoid
    D. exfoliated

27. All of the following are factors in carcinogenesis EXCEPT:
    A. heredity
    B. environment
    C. hormones
    D. bacteria

28. An example of a chromosomal disorder is
    A. cleft palate
    B. Down syndrome
    C. spina bifida
    D. anencephaly

29. A localized dilatation of an artery is called
    A. an occlusion
    B. a thrombus
    C. an aneurysm
    D. a hemorrhage

30. Malignant tumors differ from benign tumors in all the following ways EXCEPT that
    A. benign tumors do not infiltrate surrounding tissue
    B. benign tumors usually grow more quickly than malignant tumors
    C. an excised malignant tumor may recur
    D. malignant tumors set up secondary growths

31. A monogenic disorder of recessive inheritance, rare except in Jewish populations of Eastern European origin, is
    A. Klinefelter's syndrome
    B. Turner's syndrome
    C. Tay-Sachs disease
    D. Down syndrome

32. Two enzymes liberated from dying cells after a myocardial infarction are
    A. acid phosphatase and streptokinase
    B. aldactase and serum glutamic pyruvic transaminase (SGPT)
    C. creatinine phosphokinase (CPK) and serum glutamic oxaloacetic transaminase (SGOT)
    D. lactase and alkaline phosphatase

33. The congenital heart disease in which the duct joining the pulmonary artery to the aorta during intrauterine life does not become closed is
    A. tetralogy of Fallot
    B. patent ductus arteriosus
    C. coarctation of the aorta
    D. rheumatic fever

34. A patient who has edema associated with CHF would be prescribed what classification of drug?
    A. anticoagulant
    B. antibiotic

C. diuretic

D. antihypertensive

35. A patient with congestive heart failure will not demonstrate which of the following signs?

A. dyspnea

B. cyanosis

C. polycythemia

D. edema

36. A thrombotic disease of the leg vessels that occurs chiefly in young men is

A. polyarteritis nodosa

B. disseminated lupus erythematosus

C. aneurysm

D. thromboangiitis obliterans

37. A common occupational disease that afflicts gold and coal miners is

A. emphysema

B. silicosis

C. pulmonary tuberculosis

D. pneumonia

38. The most common type of lung carcinoma is

A. oat cell

B. small cell

C. squamous

D. alveolar cell

39. Achlorhydria might indicate

A. duodenal ulcer or gastritis

B. chronic dyspepsia and peptic ulcer

C. pernicious anemia and stomach cancer

D. gastric hemorrhage and duodenal ulcer

40. A disease of the stomach whose complications include hemorrhage, perforation, penetration into the pancreas, fistula formation, and obstruction is

A. gastritis

B. peptic ulcer

C. stomach cancer

D. pyloric obstruction

41. A protrusion of the intestinal mucosa and submucosa through the muscular layer is called a (an)

A. melena

B. diverticulum

C. ulcer

D. reflux

42. An acute inflammation of the colon with profuse and painful diarrhea and stools containing mucus, pus, and blood is the result of

A. typhoid fever

B. dysentery

C. ulcers

D. Crohn's disease

43. A condition in which fibrinous exudate glues the coils of the bowel together and a large amount of fluid collects in the abdominal cavity is

A. Crohn's disease

B. malabsorption syndrome

C. polyposis

D. peritonitis

44. Which of the following does not cause intestinal obstruction?

A. intussusception

B. volvulus

C. paralytic ileus

D. malabsorption syndrome

45. Icterus is caused by

A. excess bile pigment circulated in the serum

B. pyloric obstruction

C. diverticulosis

D. inadequate digestion of fats

46. When liver cells necrotize and fibrose, the condition in the liver is referred to as
    A. fibrosis
    B. cirrhosis
    C. hepatitis
    D. atrophy

47. A normal function of the gallbladder is to
    A. add liquid to the bile
    B. eliminate salts from the bile
    C. concentrate the bile
    D. excrete bile into the hepatic duct

48. Diabetes mellitus affects the body's use of fats because
    A. insulin is necessary for the combustion of fats
    B. a certain amount of carbohydrates has to be burned along with the fats when they are converted to energy
    C. low insulin levels restrict the transport of fats across cell membranes
    D. the production of ketone bodies restricts fat catabolism

49. The following are true of cystic fibrosis EXCEPT:
    A. the disease is also called mucoviscidosis
    B. the disease is familial
    C. the sweat glands are involved
    D. benign tumors of the pancreas are a feature of the disease

50. Possible signs and symptoms of diabetes mellitus include all of the following EXCEPT:
    A. glycosuria and polydipsia
    B. hyperglycemia and ketonuria
    C. air hunger and coma
    D. pancreatitis

51. The clinical picture of puffy eyes, headache, pain in the lumbar region, and small amounts of dark urine is indicative of which kidney disease?
    A. Glomerulonephritis
    B. Pyelonephritis
    C. Interstitial nephritis
    D. Nephrotic syndrome

52. Wilms' tumor is a
    A. benign tumor of the kidney
    B. malignant tumor of the kidney
    C. benign tumor of the liver
    D. malignant tumor of the liver

53. When significant amounts of kidney tissue have been destroyed by infection, vascular disease, or glomerulonephritis, the loss of the ability to excrete nitrogen-containing compounds leads to an increase in all of the following in the blood EXCEPT:
    A. urea
    B. uric acid
    C. calcium
    D. creatinine

54. When a fertilized ovum implants outside the endometrial cavity, the condition is called
    A. hydatidiform mole
    B. abruptio placenta
    C. ectopic pregnancy
    D. placenta previa

55. The correct name for fibroids is
    A. leiomyomas
    B. adenomyosis
    C. endometrial polyps
    D. endometriosis

56. All of the following are trophoblastic diseases EXCEPT:
    A. hydatidiform mole
    B. invasive mole
    C. abruptio placenta
    D. choriocarcinoma

57. The type of abortion in which the fetus dies but is retained in the uterus is a
    A. missed abortion
    B. incomplete abortion
    C. threatened abortion
    D. therapeutic abortion

58. Galactorrhea is caused by
    A. overproduction of prolactin
    B. overproduction of adrenocorticotropin
    C. underproduction of antidiuretic hormone (ADH)
    D. underproduction of prolactin

59. Adrenal cortical insufficiency is called
    A. pheochromocytoma
    B. Addison's disease
    C. myxedema
    D. Graves' disease

60. An abnormally low platelet count is termed
    A. thrombocytopenia
    B. secondary polycythemia
    C. hemolytic disease
    D. hemophilia

61. A true or primary increase in the number of red blood cells is
    A. polycythemia vera
    B. petechiae
    C. acute leukemia
    D. infectious mononucleosis

62. A disorder of the reticuloendothelial system whose symptoms include nonspecific malaise, fever, anorexia, enlarged lymph nodes, itching of the skin, and bone pain following alcohol intake is
    A. hemophilia
    B. chronic myelocytic leukemia
    C. Hodgkin's disease
    D. agranulocytosis

63. All of the following are examples of neuroses EXCEPT:
    A. anxiety
    B. senile dementia
    C. depression
    D. phobia

64. Causes of cerebral vascular accidents include all of the following EXCEPT:
    A. ischemia due to thrombosis
    B. ischemia due to embolism
    C. cerebral hemorrhage
    D. extradural hemorrhage

65. The following are all viral diseases that affect the central nervous system EXCEPT:
    A. poliomyelitis
    B. meningitis
    C. encephalitis
    D. shingles

66. A nervous system disorder marked by intention tremor, stiff gait, jerky eye movements, and a peculiar staccato speech is
    A. multiple sclerosis
    B. poliomyelitis
    C. tabes dorsalis
    D. Parkinson's disease

67. Normal cerebrospinal fluid is
    A. clear and colorless
    B. yellowish and watery
    C. waxy and clear
    D. milky in color

68. A nonbacterial disease resulting in the flattening of the head of the femur is
    A. Perthes' disease
    B. Pott's disease
    C. tuberculosis of the femur
    D. Paget's disease

69. A benign tumor of the long bones, usually in children and young adults, is
    A. osteogenic sarcoma
    B. Ewing's tumor
    C. chondroma
    D. giant cell tumor

70. Decalcification of bone due to hyperparathyroidism is
    A. rickets
    B. osteitis fibrosa cystica
    C. Paget's disease
    D. fibrous dysplasia

71. The cause of essential hypertension is
    A. chronic nephritis
    B. tumor of the adrenal cortex
    C. secondary hypertension
    D. not known

72. Immunity against diphtheria and tetanus is achieved through the injection of a (an)
    A. antibiotic
    B. exotoxin
    C. endotoxin
    D. toxoid

73. A patient who is hypokalemic would be prescribed which of the following?
    A. folic acid supplement
    B. potassium supplement
    C. iron supplement
    D. calcium supplement

74. Beginning at the stomach and continuing caudally, which is the correct sequence of intestinal parts?
    A. Duodenum, cecum, ileum, rectum
    B. Duodenum, sigmoid, appendix, anus
    C. Jejunum, ileum, cecum, sigmoid
    D. Ileum, jejunum, sigmoid, anus

75. After severe injury by trauma or after severe burns, the patient may show
    A. oliguria for several weeks
    B. anuria or oliguria for several weeks
    C. anuria or oliguria 24 to 48 hours after the injury or burn
    D. anuria for 3 to 5 days after the injury or burn

76. Prevalence of disease is the
    A. observation of the occurrence of disease in populations
    B. number of new cases of a disease per unit of time
    C. number of cases of a disease in a given population
    D. study of populations

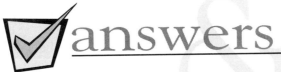

answers & rationales

1.

C. Anoxia is the sudden loss of the supply of oxygen and is the cause of cellular death after infarction. Caseation is a form of necrosis in which tissue is changed into a mass resembling cheese. Necrosis is the local death of cells, which might be caused by infarction (Sheldon, p. 47).

2.

A. Homeostasis, the balance of electrolytes and water that serves to maintain the constancy of the body's internal environment, is maintained through activity of the kidneys, lungs, liver, and the pituitary and adrenal glands (Sheldon, p. 25).

3.

A. Epidemiology gives attention not only to the cause of disease but also to the habits and characteristics of the people affected (Sheldon, p. 58).

4.

A. Vitamins B and C are water soluble. The student should know what diseases are caused by vitamin deficiencies and the major action of each vitamin in the body (Sheldon, pp. 75–77).

5.

C. Many cancers are idiopathic, as are ulcerative colitis and rheumatoid arthritis (Sheldon, p. 67).

6.

C. Physical signs are elicited by physical examination of the patient. Physical findings are synonymous with signs. Lesions are structural changes in the body caused by disease (Sheldon, p. 68).

7.

B. Dehydration occurs when there is an insufficient supply of body fluid or when body fluid is withdrawn too quickly. Effusion is the accumulation of body fluid in a compartment such as the pericardial sac or the pleural space. Ascites occurs when fluid accumulates in the peritoneal cavity (Sheldon, p. 25).

8.

D. Emboli may be due to a detached thrombus, a crushing injury to a bone (fat embolism), entrance of air into the veins (air embolism), or other causes (Sheldon, p. 91).

9.

C. Respiratory alkalosis results from a carbon dioxide deficit, usually caused by very rapid breathing, high altitudes, or heart disease. Respiratory failure is the inability of the respiratory system to maintain normal arterial gas tensions of either oxygen or carbon dioxide. Pneumonia is a lung disease of bacterial or viral origin (Sheldon, p. 106).

10.

D. First-degree burns cause only a slight reddening of the skin. Loss of blood volume (as in trauma) is called hypovolemic shock. Vasodilation allows arterioles and capillaries to become leaky; anaphylactic or severe allergic shock is of this type. Septic shock occurs with severe infections, particularly those caused by gram-negative bacteria. A fourth cause of shock is failure of the heart to pump blood (as in myocardial infarction) (Sheldon, p. 101).

11.

A. Streptococci also cause erysipelas, impetigo, and rheumatic fever (Sheldon, p. 163).

12.

A. The standard lesion of tuberculosis is the tubercle; the question outlines the stages of change that occur in the center of each tubercle (Sheldon, p. 188).

13.

C. Chancre is the primary lesion of syphilis, caused by *Treponema pallidum* (Sheldon, p. 178).

14.

D. *Candida,* commonly present on mucous membranes and in the gastrointestinal tract, can cause white patches that, when occurring in the mouth, are called thrush (Sheldon, p. 232).

15.

B. Trematodes include flukes; the most common disease they cause is schistosomiasis. Trypanosomes cause sleeping sickness. Pediculi are lice (Sheldon, p. 235).

16.

A. When the cut margins of a wound are brought together by adhesive bandage, suture, or pressure, it is called healing by first intention. In healing by second intention, the cut margins are not brought together (answer C) (Sheldon, p. 123).

17.

B. Antigens are substances that, in the body, provoke the immune response to which an antibody reacts specifically. T cells and B cells are two kinds of lymphocytes (Sheldon, pp. 128–131).

18.

A. The other three answers are fabrications. Hypersensitivity is an increase in sensitivity to a particular antigen or an abnormal overreaction by an oversensitive immune system (Sheldon, pp. 138–139).

19.

A. Coumadin is an anticoagulant and therefore would be used for the treatment of venous thrombosis (Spratto & Woods, p. 1369).

20.

C. Cholera causes excessive fluid loss from diarrhea. The resulting dehydration causes death in 75% of cases (Sheldon, p. 170).

21.

B. Ringworm of the scalp (tinea), ringworm of the groin, and interdigital ringworm (athlete's foot) are three dermatomycoses (Sheldon, p. 233).

22.

D. Angiomas are composed of vessels, usually blood vessels but also lymph vessels. A common site is the skin, where the angioma is often called a port-wine stain or birthmark. Other benign tumors include adenomas, lipomas, leiomyomas, and nevi (Sheldon, p. 262).

23.

C. Tuberculosis is caused by an acid-fast bacillus, *Mycobacterium tuberculosis.* Leprosy is also caused by an acid-fast bacillus, *Mycobacterium leprae.* Diphtheria is caused by a gram-positive bacillus, *Corynebacterium diphtheriae.* Gonorrhea is caused by a gram-negative coccus, *Neisseria gonorrhoeae.* Botulism, caused by *Clostridium botulinum,* tetanus (*Clostridium tetani*), and gas gangrene (*Clostridium perfringens*) are all gram-positive bacilli and are anaerobes. Typhoid fever is caused by a gram-negative rod, *Salmonella typhi.* All of these are aerobes (Sheldon, pp. 175–176).

24.

B. Erysipelas is an inflammation of the lymphatics of the skin. Legionnaire's disease is a respiratory illness. Rheumatic fever's most striking clinical feature is acute inflammation of the joints (Sheldon, p. 173).

25.

D. Tetanus is caused by an anaerobic bacterium. All the other conditions listed are caused by viruses (Sheldon, pp. 196–225).

26.

A. Anaplastic tumors are also called undifferentiated. They are usually highly malignant (Sheldon, p. 263).

27.

D. Other factors include chemical carcinogens, ionizing radiation, viruses, and chronic irritation (Sheldon, pp. 251–259).

28.

B. Spina bifida and anencephaly are considered congenital malformations rather than inherited diseases. Cleft palate is a multifactorial birth defect that develops from the interaction of many factors (Sheldon, pp. 271–272).

29.

C. All aneurysms are due to weakening of the arterial wall and are usually due to atherosclerosis (Sheldon, p. 331).

30.

B. Malignant tumors usually grow more quickly than benign tumors. Secondary growths from primary malignant tumors (answer D) are called metastases (Sheldon, p. 260).

31.

C. The other three are chromosomal disorders in which there are abnormalities in the structure or number of chromosomes (Sheldon, pp. 287–288).

32.

C. CPK and SGOT may rise from 2 to 20 times normal, 24 hours after an infarction (Sheldon, p. 296).

33.

B. Tetralogy of Fallot results in pulmonary valve stenosis, ventricular septal defect, right ventricular hypertrophy, and the aorta overriding the right ventricle. Coarctation of the aorta is a narrowing of the aorta. Rheumatic fever is not a congenital disease but a bacterial disease of the joints and heart (Sheldon, p. 303).

34.

C. Diuretics such as Lasix would be used to treat edema, cyanosis, or any type of accumulation of fluids in the body (Spratto & Woods, p. 660).

35.

C. Dyspnea is the most common symptom of heart failure causing cyanosis. Edema is most marked in the hands and feet. Polycythemia (increased number of red blood cells) is a common feature of congenital heart disease (Sheldon, p. 11).

36.

D. Polyarteritis nodosa is an inflammatory collagen disease involving the small arteries of the viscera. Disseminated lupus erythematosus is also a collagen disease and is distinguished by a butterfly rash over the bridge of the nose and cheeks. An aneurysm is a localized dilatation of an artery (Sheldon, p. 330).

37.

B. Silicosis arises from inhalation of dust containing silica. Emphysema is characterized by an increase in the volume of the lung. Pulmonary tuberculosis is caused by a bacillus (a bacterium), while pneumonia can be bacterial or viral in origin (Sheldon, p. 352).

38.

C. Oat cell and small cell carcinoma of the lung are the same disease and account for about 15% of all lung cancers. Alveolar cell carcinoma accounts for about 3% and squamous cell cancer for about 40% (Sheldon, p. 351).

39.

C. There is a high incidence of adenocarcinoma of the stomach with little or no hydrochloric acid. Pernicious anemia is a disease of the bone marrow and hematopoietic (blood-forming) system and is due to the lack of a stomach secretion (intrinsic factor) that is responsible for the absorption of vitamin B_{12} (Sheldon, pp. 365–366).

40.

B. The most serious complication of gastritis is bleeding. Pyloric obstruction is a common result of stomach cancer (Sheldon, pp. 366–368).

41.

B. The presence of diverticula in large numbers is termed diverticulosis. If a diverticulum becomes inflamed, the condition is called diverticulitis (Sheldon, pp. 379–380).

42.

B. The two kinds of dysentery are amebic (caused by *Entamoeba histolytica*) and bacillary (caused by *Shigella* bacilli) (Sheldon, p. 378).

43.

D. Peritonitis is inflammation of the thin membrane that lines the abdominal cavity. The usual cause is a ruptured appendix (Sheldon, p. 378).

44.

D. Malabsorption syndromes are characterized by diarrhea and abnormal bowel movements. There are several causes, including adult sprue and diseases of the pancreas and liver (Sheldon, pp. 375–376).

45.

A. Three types of jaundice are hemolytic, obstructive, and hepatocellular (Sheldon, pp. 386–389).

46.

B. Cirrhosis is a morphological response to continuing injury to the liver (Sheldon, pp. 397–400).

47.

C. When the gallbladder has been inflamed repeatedly due to chemical (acute cholecystitis), mechanical (gallstones), or infectious irritation, the ability to concentrate bile is impaired (Sheldon, p. 403).

48.

B. Although diabetes mellitus initially involves a derangement of carbohydrate metabolism, the resulting disorders in fat metabolism lead to death if unchecked (Sheldon, p. 412).

49.

D. Benign adenomas of the pancreas (beta cell tumors and alpha tumors) may result in death if the correct diagnosis is not made (Sheldon, p. 420).

50.

D. All of the symptoms and signs listed can be manifested in diabetes mellitus except pancreatitis (Sheldon, p. 416).

51.

A. Glomerulonephritis often occurs as a sequel to acute ear infections or scarlet fever (Sheldon, pp. 427–428).

52.

B. Wilms' tumor occurs in children, usually during the first 3 years of life (Sheldon, pp. 432–433).

53.

C. The result is uremia. Hypercalcemia is due 95% of the time to hyperparathyroid disease. Also, calcium is not a nitrogen-containing compound, as are the other three answers (Sheldon, pp. 429–430).

54.

C. Implantation usually occurs in the fallopian tube. Abruptio placenta occurs when a portion of the placenta separates from the implantation site prematurely. Placenta previa is insertion of the placenta near or covering the cervical canal (Sheldon, p. 458).

55.

A. These tumors are composed of smooth muscle tissue rather than fibrous tissue (Sheldon, p. 453).

56.

C. Trophoblasts are the cells of the placenta. Hydatidiform mole is an abnormal product of conception in which there is usually no fetus. It may represent the missed abortion of a blighted ovum. An invasive mole is one in which molar tissue is found deep in the myometrium. Choriocarcinoma is a malignant tumor of the trophoblast (Sheldon, pp. 460–461).

57.

A. Missed, threatened, and incomplete abortions are examples of spontaneous abortions. Therapeutic abortions are performed when a pregnancy endangers the mother's mental or physical health (Sheldon, p. 459; Taber's, p. 7).

58.

A. Galactorrhea is milk secretion without pregnancy. Overproduction of adrenocorticotropin (ACTH) causes Cushing's syndrome. Underproduction of ADH causes diabetes insipidus (Sheldon, p. 473).

59.

B. Pheochromocytoma is a tumor of the adrenal medulla. Myxedema is adult hypothyroidism. Graves' disease (toxic diffuse goiter) is the most common cause of excess circulating thyroid hormone (Sheldon, p. 477).

60.

A. Thrombocytopenia often leads to bleeding; there are several causes (Sheldon, p. 504).

61.

A. Petechiae are small hemorrhages in the skin and may appear when platelets are decreased in number (thrombocytopenia). Acute leukemia is indicated most commonly by an episode of hemorrhage (nosebleed, etc.) in an otherwise normal child. Infectious mononucleosis is characterized by a sore throat, fever, swollen lymph nodes, and lassitude (Sheldon, p. 503).

62.

C. None of the other diseases listed is of the reticuloendothelial system, and all have different symptoms (Sheldon, p. 513).

63.

B. Sheldon defines neuroses as "all those mental disorders that have no demonstrable organic basis, and in which the patient may have considerable insight and unimpaired reality testing." Senile dementia has an organic basis (Sheldon, pp. 517–518).

64.

D. Extradural hemorrhage occurs when blood pours out between the skull and the dura mater but does not enter the brain tissue (Sheldon, pp. 519–522).

65.

B. Meningitis is a bacterial infection. Shingles is the common name for herpes zoster (Sheldon, pp. 529–530).

66.

A. Parkinson's disease is characterized by rigidity of involuntary muscles, tremor of fingers and hands, and an attitude of flexion throughout the body. Tabes dorsalis is a syphilitic disease of the spinal cord and involves loss of muscular coordination of the legs. Poliomyelitis, if the infection becomes clinically apparent, results in paralysis (Sheldon, pp. 531–532).

67.

A. Cerebrospinal fluid contains sugar and chlorides, but no proteins (Sheldon, p. 539).

68.

A. In Perthes' (or Legg-Perthes') disease, the aseptic lesion is confined to the head of the femur, representing aseptic necrosis of the bone due to ischemia. Pott's disease is tuberculosis of the spine, and Paget's disease, or osteitis deformans, shows an increase in bone cell activity resulting in structural deformities (Sheldon, p. 557).

69.

D. Ewing's tumor is a malignant tumor that profusely involves several bones and appears mainly between the ages of 5 and 15. Chondroma is a benign tumor of cartilage. Osteogenic sarcoma occurs at the end of long bones, especially in the region of the knee (Sheldon, p. 542).

70.

B. This disease is also called von Recklinghausen's disease and is characterized by highly porous and decalcified bones (Sheldon, p. 561).

71.

D. Chronic nephritis and tumor of the adrenal cortex are both associated with secondary hypertension.

Other conditions, especially of the kidney and adrenal glands, are also associated with secondary hypertension (Sheldon, p. 98).

72.

D. Toxins, in this sense, are the poisons produced by bacteria. An exotoxin is a poison, secreted by living bacteria, that occurs in diphtheria, gas gangrene, and botulism. An exotoxin treated with formaldehyde confers immunity rather than causing the disease; this modified bacterium is called a toxoid. An endotoxin is liberated when bacteria die and disintegrate. An antibiotic fights an infection that is already present but it does not confer immunity (Sheldon, p. 157).

73.

B. Hypokalemia would be treated with an oral potassium supplement (Dorland's, p. 401).

74.

C. The jejunum and ileum are parts of the small intestine; the cecum and sigmoid are parts of the large intestine (Sheldon, p. 372).

75.

C. Shock following the injury causes necrosis of the proximal convoluted tubules; it is reversible in a large percentage of cases (Sheldon, pp. 428–429).

76.

C. Answer A is a definition of epidemiology; answer B is a definition of incidence of disease; answer D is a definition of demography (Sheldon, p. 55).

References

2000 Accel-Team.Com. (2002). *Job enlargement and job enrichment. Factoring in Herzberg's two factor theory of motivation* [Online]. Retrieved November 15, 2002, from http://www.accel-team.com/work_design/wd_02.html

Abdelhak, M., Grostick, S., Hanken, M., & Jacobs, E. (2001). *HEALTH INFORMATION: Management of a strategic resource (2nd ed.)*. Philadelphia: W.B. Saunders.

Bernstein, J. (2002). *Crisis management, response, prevention, planning and training* [Online]. Retrieved November 13, 2002, from http://bernstein.com/nl/crisismgr.000215.html

Brown, F. (2002). *ICD-9-CM coding handbook, with answers.* Chicago: American Hospital Association.

Buck, C. (2002). *Hospital and Payor ICD-9-CM, Volumes 1, 2, & 3 and HCPCS Level II.* Philadelphia: W.B. Saunders.

Buck, C. (2002). *Step-by-step medical coding.* Philadelphia: W.B. Saunders.

CMS. (2002). *Computer-based training—Medicare fraud and abuse* [Online]. Retrieved October 19, 2002, from http://www.cms.hhs.gov/medlearn/CBT_frau.asp

Cofer, J., & Greeley, H. (1998). *Continuous quality for health information management.* MA: Opus Communications.

Current Procedural Terminology (4th ed.) (2003). Chicago: American Medical Association.

Fordney, F., & French, L. (2003). *Medical insurance billing and coding: An essentials worktext.* Philadelphia: W.B. Saunders.

Freedman, A. (2001). *Computer desktop encyclopedia (9th ed.).* Berkeley, CA: Obsborne/McGraw Hill.

Glondys, B. (1999). *Documentation guidelines for the acute care patient record.* Chicago: American Health Information Management Association.

Healey JF. (1984). *Statistics: A tool for social research.* Belmont, CA: Wadsworth.

Health Forum. (2002). *AHA guide to the health care field 2002–2003* [Online]. Retrieved November 15, 2002, from http://www.aha.org

Huffman, E. (1994). *Health information management (10th ed.).* Berwyn, IL: Physicians' Record Company.

Johns, M. (2002). *Health information management technology*. Chicago: American Health Information Management Association.

Koch, G. (1996). *Basic allied health statistics and analysis*. Albany, NY: Delmar.

Mattingly R. (1997). *Management of health information, functions and applications*. Albany, NY: Delmar.

McDonnel-Brown, G. (1990). *The art of leadership—Managerial grid* [Online]. Retrieved November 15, 2002, from http://home.iprimus.com.an/bill58/leadership.htm

Motley, N. (2002). *Federal regulations and nursing homes* [Online]. Retrieved November 16, 2002, from http://www.nursinghomealert.com/stoppingabuse/federalregulations.html

NetMBA Business Knowledge Center. (2002). *Theory X and Theory Y* [Online]. Retrieved November 14, 2002, from http://www.netmba.com/mgmt/ob/motivation/mcgregor

Norwood, G. (2002). *Maslow hierarchy of needs* [Online]. Retrieved November 14, 2002, from http://www.connect.net/georgen/maslow.htm

Peden, A. (1998). *Comparative records for health information management*. Albany, NY: Delmar.

Reh, F. (2002). *Management feature: Managing the talent pool* [Online]. Retrieved November 13, 2002, from http://lad.doubleclick.net/adi/abt.smallbusiness/smallbusiness_managmeent;svc=;site=management/html

RHIA/RHIT Certification Guide [Online]. (2001). AHIMA. Retrieved September 20, 2002, from www.ahima.org

Sheldon, H. (1992). *Boyd's introduction to the study of disease (11th ed.)*. Philadelphia: Lippincott Williams & Wilkins.

Smith, G. (2002). *Basic CPT/HCPCS coding*. Chicago: American Health Information Management Association.

Social Security Online. (2002). *Social Security online*. Retrieved November 14, 2002, from http://www.ssa.gov/

Spratto, G. (2002). *PDR nurse's drug handbook (2002 ed.)*. Montvale, NJ: Delmar.

Stedman's medical dictionary (27th ed.). Philadelphia: Lippincott Willliams & Wilkins.

Stuart-Kotze, A. (2002). *Four classic motivation theories* [Online]. Retrieved November 14, 2002, from www.managementlearning.com

Symmetry Software Corporation. (2002). *Fringe benefits* [Online]. Retrieved November 15, 2002, from http://payroll-taxes.com/default.htm

Taber's cyclopedic medical dictionary. (18th ed.). (1997). Philadelphia: F.A. Davis.

U.S. Department of Health and Human Services, Centers for Medicare and Medicaid Services. (2002) *Medicare & You 2003* [Online]. Retrieved September 15, 2002, from http://www.medicare.gov/publications/pubs/pdf/10050.pdf.

West's Encyclopedia of American Law. (2002). *Unemployment compensation* [Online]. Retrieved November 14, 2002, from http://www.wld.com/conbus/weal/wunemp.html

Youmans, K. (2000). *Basic healthcare statistics for health information management professionals*. Chicago: American Health Information Management Association.

Index

A

Abortion, 195, 201
Accession registries, 10, 18
Accident reports, 24, 32
Accreditation, 23, 32
Accreditation Manual, 95, 102
Accreditation surveys, 20, 28
Accreditation with commendation, 23, 31
Achlorhydria, 193, 200
Active staff members, 23, 31
Activities of daily living, 56, 62
Adrenal cortical insufficiency, 195, 201
Affirmative action, 177, 185
Alphabetical filing, 7, 16
Ambulatory care, 20–23, 25, 28–30, 33
American College of Surgeons, 2, 11
Anaerobic bacterial diseases, 191, 198
Anaplastic tumors, 192, 199
Ancillary departments, 6, 15
Anesthesiologists, 21, 29
Aneurysms, 192, 199
Annual reports, 7, 16
Anoxia, 190, 197
APACHE II, 41, 49
Assault, 113, 119
Asterisks, 37, 46
ASTM E1384, 21, 29
Authority, 178, 186
Autopsy rates, 94, 98, 101, 105
Autopsy reports, 8, 17
Average length of stay, 94, 101

B

Balanced Budget Act of 1997, 57, 63
Bar coding, 5, 15
Bar graphs, 99, 107
Battery, 113, 119
Bed counts, 96, 103
Bed turnover rates, 94, 101–2
Best evidence rule, 116, 122
Bills of particulars, 113, 119–20
Biomedical sciences, 189–202

Birth certificates, 6, 15
Budgeting, 153–54, 156–57, 159, 163–167
Burns, 42, 50, 190, 196, 197–98, 202
Bylaws, 22, 30

C

Cancer registries, 5, 10, 14, 18
Candida, 191, 198
Capitation, 58, 64
Carcinogenesis, 192, 199
Case eligibility data, 10, 18
Case finding, 10, 18
Case-mix systems, 56, 62
Census, 95, 102
Centers for Medicare and Medicaid Services, 56, 62
Certification, 23, 32
Certification of Compliance, 116, 122
CHAMPVA, 58, 63–64
Chancres, 191, 198
Charge capture, 127, 133
Chargemaster forms, 59, 64
Check sheets, 143, 149
Chief complaints, 4, 6, 9, 13, 15, 17
Cholera, 191, 198
Chromosomal disorders, 192, 199
Cirrhosis, 194, 200
Classification systems, 35–53
Client-server technology, 125, 132
Clinical pathways, 144, 150
Coding, 34–53
　　CPT-4, 67–92
　　diagnosis, 36, 46
　　IDC-9-CM, 67–92
Color coding, 4, 13
Community care, 20, 28
Comorbidity, 42, 50
Compliance program guidance, 57, 63
Complications, 37, 46
Confidentiality, 24, 32, 126, 133
Congestive heart failure, 193, 199

Consent, 112–13, 114, 115, 119, 120, 121
Consulting staff members, 23, 31
Correct Coding Initiative (CCI), 57, 58, 63
Cost control, 22–23, 30
Coumadin, 191, 198
CPT-4 coding, 67–92
Cystic fibrosis, 194, 200

D

Daily analysis of hospital service, 95, 102
Daily census, 96, 97, 103, 104–5
Data, 124, 131. See also Information technology
　　content and structure of, 1–18
　　literacy, 93–108
　　validity of, 96, 103
Dead on arrival (DOA), 94, 101
Death certificates, 6, 15
Death rates, 97, 104
　　gross, 94–95, 96, 98, 102, 103, 105
　　net, 94–95, 102
Decalcification, 196, 202
Defamation, 115, 121
Deficiency analysis, 6, 15
Dehydration, 190, 197
DHHS, 96, 103
Diabetes mellitus, 194, 200
Diagnosis. See also Coding
　　primary, 4, 13
　　principal, 4, 13, 59, 60, 64, 65
　　provisional, 4, 13
Diagnostic related groups, 56, 59, 60, 62, 64, 65
Dictation systems, 126, 128, 132, 134
Discharge summaries, 2–3, 11, 24, 32
Discrimination, 175, 176, 183, 185
Disease indexes, 7, 16
Disease staging, 41, 49
Dislocations, 42, 50
Diuretics, 192–93, 199
Diverticulum, 193, 200

Divorce, 3, 12
DRG grouping, 41, 49, 56–57, 62
DSM-IV, 40, 48
Dysentery, 193, 200

E

Ectopic pregnancy, 194, 201
E-mail, 124, 131
Emboli, 190, 197
Emergency patients, 6, 15
Employee assistant programs (EAPs), 172, 181
Employee evaluations, 174, 179, 182–83, 187
Employers, information to, 110, 117
Encounters, 22, 30
Epidemiology, 190, 196, 197, 202
Eponyms, 38, 47
Error rates, 140, 146
Errors, 8, 17
    correcting, 2, 11
    dosage, 41, 49
Erysipelas, 192, 199
Ethernet, 125, 132
Ethical issues, 109–22
Ewing's tumor, 196, 202
Exempt employees, 177, 185
Explanations of benefits (EOBs), 58, 64

F

Fair Labor Standards Act, 172, 178, 181, 186
Family numbering systems, 9, 17
Fat-soluble vitamins, 190, 197
Federal Register, 115, 121
Fetal deaths, 94, 97, 101, 104
Fibroids, 194, 201
File guides, 9, 18
Filing, 125, 132. *See also* Information technology; Numbering systems
    alphabetical order in, 3, 12
    color coding in, 4, 13
Fiscal intermediaries, 58, 63
Flextime, 172, 181
Foreign bodies, 42, 50
Forms
    designing, 6, 15
    revising, 24, 32
Fractures, 39, 42, 48, 50

G

Glalactorrhea, 195, 201
Glomerulonephritis, 194, 200
Glossary of Health Care Terms, 95, 102
Governing boards, 25, 33
Graphs, 99, 100, 106–7, 142, 148–49, 154, 163. *See also* Statistics

Grievances, 174, 177, 183, 185
Gross death rates, 94–95, 96, 98, 102, 103, 105
Group practices, 21, 29
Guide to the Health Care Field, 95, 102

H

Hazard surveillance checklists, 140, 146–147
HCFA 1500, 57, 63
Healing by first intention, 191, 198
Health care delivery systems, 19–34
Health maintenance organizations (HMOs), 20, 23, 28, 30–31
Hearsay evidence, 113, 119
Hierarchy of needs, 178, 186
History reports, 4, 13
Home health care, 24–25, 25, 32–33, 33
    plans of care in, 27, 35
Homeostasis, 190, 197
Honorary staff members, 23, 31
Hospice programs, 20, 21, 23, 28, 29, 31
Hospital administration, 20, 28
Human resources, 171–88
Hypersensitivity, 191, 198
Hypertension, 196, 202
Hypokalemia, 196, 202

I

ICD-9-CM coding, 67–92
Icterus, 193, 200
Idiopathic disease, 190, 197
Immune response, 191, 198
Incidence, 196, 202
Incident reports, 5, 14, 24, 32, 112, 118, 139, 146
Incomplete records, 8, 10, 16, 17, 18
Independent practice associations, 24, 32
Infants
    low birth weight, 94, 95, 101, 102
    records of, 5, 14, 94, 101
Information, 124, 131. *See also* Data; Information technology
Information technology, 123–36
Inpatient admissions, 97, 104
Inpatient records, 4, 13
Inpatient service days, 94, 101
Insurance claims, 57, 63
Integrated health record format, 2, 11, 23, 31

J

Jaundice, 193, 200
JCAHO, 4, 6, 9, 10, 13, 15, 18, 23, 31
Job descriptions, 152, 155, 162, 164, 175, 184

Job enlargement, 178, 186
Job enrichment, 173, 182

L

Lawsuits, 110, 117
Layout planning, 152, 158, 160, 162, 166, 168
Leadership, 156–57, 165
Leaves of absence, 95, 102
Legal issues, 109–22
Length of stay, 97, 104
Liability, 116, 122, 138, 145
Libel, 115, 121
Line graphs, 100, 107
Local area networks, 127, 133
Long-term care facilities, 20, 23, 24, 26, 28, 31, 32, 34
    case-mix system in, 41, 49
Low birth weight neonates, 94, 95, 101, 102
Lung carcinomas, 193, 200

M

Malabsorption syndromes, 193, 200
Malignant tumors, 191, 192, 198, 199
Manipulation/reduction, 39, 48
Master patient indexes
    retention of, 3, 12
Medicaid, 59, 64
Medicare, 58, 59, 61, 63, 64, 66, 127, 133
    fraud/abuse, 56, 62
    prospective payment system, 57, 63
    quality management and, 141, 147
Mental health care facilities, 25, 26, 33
Methods improvement, 172, 182
Microfilming, 3, 5, 7, 12, 14, 16, 110, 117, 159, 167
Minimum contents standards, 4, 13
Minimum d43,51, 42, 50
Minimum data sets, 24, 32
Minors, 114, 116, 120, 122
Motivation, 172, 181
Movement diagrams, 177, 185
Multihospital systems, 25, 33
Municipally owned hospitals, 21, 30
Myocardial infarction, 192, 199

N

NEC (not elsewhere classifiable), 37, 47
Negligence, 115, 121
Neighborhood health centers, 25, 33
Neoplasm Table, 41, 49
Net death rates, 94–95, 102
Neuroses, 195, 201
Nomenclature, 36, 46
NOS, 36, 46
Null hypothesis, 142, 148
Number indexes, 8, 16–17

Numbering systems, 9, 17. *See also* Filing
  divorce and, 3, 12
  purging and, 3, 12
  straight numeric, 5, 14
Nursing facilities, 23, 31

O

Occasions of service, 22, 30
Occupancy, percent of, 94, 97, 98, 101, 104, 105
Occupational Safety and Health Administration (OSHA), 174, 183
Occurrence screening, 140, 147
Omit code, 40, 48
Omnibus Budget Reconciliation Act of 1990 (OBRA), 56, 62
Operational plans, 157, 166
Ophthalmologists, 21, 29
Optometrists, 21, 29
Organization/supervision, 151–59
OSHA, 174, 183
Osteopaths, 21, 25, 29, 33
Outpatient visits, 22, 30
Output devices, 127, 133
Overutilization, 141, 147

P

Parentheses, 38, 47
Pathology reports, 8, 17
Patient registers, 5, 14
Pay systems, 174, 183
Peer review organizations, 22, 30
Peptic ulcers, 193, 200
Performance improvement, 137–50
Peritonitis, 193, 200
Personal use of records, 2, 11
Perthes' disease, 195, 202
Petechiae, 195, 201
Physical examination reports, 6, 15
Physician relocation, 20, 28
PL92-603, 143, 149
Point-of-service plans, 24, 32
Polyarteritis nodosa, 193, 199
Postanesthesia evaluations, 3, 12
Preferred provider organizations, 24, 25, 32, 33, 140, 146
Pretrial discovery, 116, 122
Prevalence, 196, 202
Primary records, 2, 11
Principal diagnosis, 59, 60, 64, 65
Principal procedures, 60, 66
Privileged communication, 110, 114, 117, 120
Problem-oriented records, 3, 7, 12, 15
  sections of, 4, 13
Procedure documents, 154, 157–58, 160, 164, 166, 168
Productivity, 153, 161, 163, 169

Progress notes, 2–3, 4, 9, 11, 13, 18
Prospective payment system, 57, 58, 60, 63, 65
PS 92-603, 139, 146
PSROs, 139, 145–46
Purging systems, 3, 12

Q

Quality assessment, 137–50
Quantitative analysis, 5, 14

R

Radiation therapy treatments, 3, 12
R-ADT (Registration-Admissions, Discharges and Transfers) systems, 127, 134
Ratios, computing, 99, 106
RBVRS (Resource Based Relative Value System), 56, 62
Reanalysis, 3, 12
Record control function, 3, 12
Record linkage, 127, 133
Record ownership, 110, 113, 117, 120
Records
  inactive, 4, 13
  incomplete, 8, 10, 16, 17, 18
  infants', 5, 14, 94, 101
  inpatient, 4, 13
  personal use of, 2, 11
  primary, 2, 11
  problem-oriented, 3, 4, 7, 12, 13, 15
  release of, 24, 26, 32, 34–35, 110–22
  retention of, 3, 12, 112, 119
  secondary patient, 114, 120
  source-oriented, 8, 16
  tampering with, 110, 117
  tracking, 125, 132
Redisclosure, 113, 120
Reengineering, 144, 150
Referral statements, 24, 32
Rehabilitative care, 20, 26, 28, 34
Reimbursement methodologies, 55–66
Relative value units (RVUs), 56, 62
Release of records, 24, 26, 32, 34–35, 110–22
Research design, 140–41, 147–48
Res ipsa loquitur, 111, 118
Resource utilization groups, 41, 49, 56, 62
Respiratory alkalosis, 190, 197
Respite care, 20, 28
Respondeat superior, 111, 118
Reviews of systems, 4, 13
Ringworm, 191, 198
Risk management programs, 138, 139, 141, 145, 146, 147
Rubber stamps, 2, 11

Rules and regulations, medical staff, 22, 30

S

Safety reviews, 138, 145
Scarlet fever, 190–91, 198
Secondary patient records, 114, 120
Security, data, 124, 128, 131, 134
Serial-unit numbering, 3, 12
Shelving, 8, 17
Signs, 190, 197
Silicosis, 193, 199–200
SOAP notes, 7, 8, 16, 17
Social security numbers, 7, 9, 16, 17
Source-oriented records, 8, 16
Space planning, 152, 158, 160, 162, 166, 168
Span of control, 179, 187
Spreadsheet software, 128, 134
Standard deviations, 99, 107
Standards of care, 112, 119
Standing orders, 6, 15
Statistics, 93–108, 137–50
Statutes of limitations, 115, 120
Strategic plans, 159, 167
Subpoenas, 110–11, 112, 113, 114, 115, 117, 118, 120
Supervision, 151–59
Surgery codes, 39, 48
Systems development life cycle (SDLC), 128–29, 135

T

Tampering with records, 110, 117
Tay-Sachs disease, 192, 199
Telephone requests for release of information, 114, 115, 120, 121
Terminal digit numbering, 3, 4, 5, 7, 12, 14, 16
Tetanus, 192, 199
Thrombocytopenia, 195, 201
Time-sharing, 125, 132
Torts, 115, 121
Toxicity, 42, 49–50
Training, 174, 183
Transfer statements, 24, 32
Trematodes, 191, 198
Trophoblastic diseases, 194, 201
T-test, 96, 103
Tuberculosis, 191, 198

U

UB-92, 60, 65
UHDDS, 60, 65, 98, 106
Unbundling, 58, 63
Unit numbering systems, 3, 7, 12, 16
Unity of command, 178, 186
Uremia, 194, 201

"Use additional code," 37, 47
Utilization management plans, 138, 145
Utilization reviews, 23, 26, 31, 34, 139, 146

V

Validity, 100, 107
Veterans Health Administration, 9, 17

W

Wilms' tumor, 194, 201
Witnesses, legal, 110, 117
Word processing software, 124, 126, 128, 131, 133, 134
Work distribution charts, 153, 155, 162, 164, 175, 178, 184, 186

Work sampling, 175, 178, 180, 184, 186, 188

Z

Zero defects, 141, 148